CLINICAL TEACHING IN CANADIAN NURSING

CANADIAN ASSOCIATION OF SCHOOLS OF NURSING

EDITORS:

SHERRI MELROSE

BETH PERRY

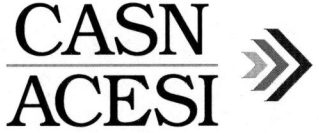

Copyright © Canadian Association Of Schools Of Nursing 2022

www.casn.ca

Clinical Teaching in Canadian Nursing

All rights reserved. No part of this publication may be reproduced, stored in a retrieval system or transmited in any form or by any means, electronic, mechanical, photocopying, recording or otherwise without the prior permision of the publisher or in accordance with the provisions of the Copyright (Canadian Copyright Agency).

Published by: Canadian Association Of Schools Of Nursing

Library and Archives Canada Cataloguing in Publication

Title: Clinical teaching in Canadian nursing / Sherri Melrose, Beth Perry, editors.
Names: Melrose, Sherri, 1951- editor. | Perry, Beth, 1957- editor. | Canadian Association of Schools of Nursing, publisher.
Description: Includes bibliographical references and index.
Identifiers: Canadiana (print) 20220146802 | Canadiana (ebook) 20220146829 | ISBN 9781989648209 (softcover) | ISBN 9781989648216 (PDF)
Subjects: LCSH: Nursing—Study and teaching. | LCSH: Clinical competence—Study and teaching.
Classification: LCC RT81.6 .C55 2022 | DDC 610.73071/1—dc23

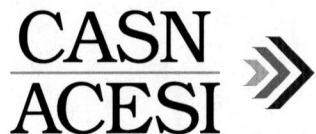

Contents

VIII	**AUTHOR BIOGRAPHIES**
1	**CHAPTER 1**
	Historical Context of Practice-Based Learning
13	**CHAPTER 2**
	The Role of the Clinical Instructor
25	**CHAPTER 3**
	Pedagogy of Clinical Teaching
40	**CHAPTER 4**
	Fostering the Development of Clinical Judgement and Reasoning

53	**CHAPTER 5**
	Practice-Based Learning in Acute Care Settings
89	**CHAPTER 6**
	Practice-Based Learning in Community Placements
115	**CHAPTER 7**
	Assessing and Evaluating Students in the Clinical Setting
134	**CHAPTER 8**
	Legal and Ethical Dimensions of Clinical Instructing
150	**APPENDIX**
153	**INDEX**

List of Figures

- Figure 1.1 Staff and First Graduating Class of the Mack Training School for Nurses
- Figure 2.1 Tuckman and Jensen's (1977) Stages of Group Development
- Figure 3.1 Bloom's Taxonomy
- Figure 4.1 Characteristics of Students' Clinical Judgement and Reasoning in a Three-Year Undergraduate Bachelor of Nursing Program
- Figure 4.2 List of Challenges and Remediation Strategies for Clinical Instructors
- Figure 5.1 List of Materials to Be Included in a Student Nurse Orientation Package
- Figure 5.2 Nursing Student Do's and Don'ts
- Figure 5.3 Skeleton Schedule
- Figure 5.4 Key Components of the Nursing Brain Sheet
- Figure 5.5 Adapted SBAR Tool
- Figure 5.6 Clinical Learning Activities for Post-Conference
- Figure 6.1 Sample Gantt Chart of Clinical Activities in a Community Placement over the Term Mapped to Course Learning Outcomes (CLOs) and Tanner's Model of Clinical Reasoning and Judgement (Community Health Nursing Process)
- Figure 7.1 A Comparison of Formative and Summative Clinical Course Evaluation
- Figure 7.2 The Clinical Evaluation Process
- Figure 7.3 Personal Clinical Learning Plan
- Figure 7.4 Examples of Comments to Support Student Learning
- Figure 7.5 Remediation Plan Example – Contract
- Figure 7.6 Clinical Evaluation Tool Example
- Figure 7.7 Sample Descriptors for Levelled Student Clinical Performance

List of Boxes

- Box 5.1 Questions Clinical Instructors Should Ask During the First Meeting with Students
- Box 8.1 Case Example
- Box 8.2 Case Example
- Box 8.3 Case Study

AUTHOR BIOGRAPHIES

Cynthia Baker

Cynthia Baker is the executive director of the Canadian Association of Schools of Nursing (CASN) and a professor emerita of Queen's University in Canada. She is the former director of Queen's University School of Nursing and associate dean of the Health Science Faculty. Before that, she was the director of l'École de science infirmière de l'Université de Moncton. Her educational qualifications include a bachelor's degree from McGill University in Canada; an MPhil in anthropology from the University of London, England; a Master of Nursing from Dalhousie University in Canada; and a PhD from the University of Texas at Austin in the United States.

Genevieve Currie

Genevieve Currie RN, MN, PhD (candidate) is an associate professor in the School of Nursing and Midwifery at Mount Royal University in Calgary, Alberta. Her nursing experience is in pediatrics, family newborn, population health, and community health nursing. Her current research and teaching interests are focused on community health nursing practice and education, family centered care, and family engagement in health care and research. Genevieve is a member of the Community Health Nurses of Canada, Leadership Standing Committee.

Marie-France Deschênes

Marie-France Deschênes is a postdoctoral fellow at the University of Ottawa (2021–2022) and an assistant professor in the Faculty of Nursing at the Université de Montréal (starting April 2022). As a nurse educator, she has extensive experience in the supervision of students in the clinical setting. Her research interests are clinical reasoning, script concordance, competence evaluation, and cognitive companionship.

Kariane Holmes

Kariane Holmes is a registered nurse currently practising in Vancouver, British Columbia, in pediatric intensive care. She previously practiced in Toronto, Ontario, on an acute pediatric cardiology inpatient unit and pediatric critical care unit, where she discovered her passion for teaching pre-service learners including nursing students, clinical externs, and new graduate nurses. Kariane's passion for education in the acute practice setting is also echoed in her previous experience with as a family education nurse for in-service learners and safety coach team lead. Kariane completed her master of nursing degree with a clinical teaching focus at Athabasca University, Alberta, Canada.

Patrick Lavoie

Patrick Lavoie is an assistant professor in the Faculty of Nursing at the Université de Montréal and a researcher at the Montreal Heart Institute, Quebec, Canada. He specializes in critical care nursing education, and his research seeks to understand and improve nurses' clinical judgement and reasoning with deteriorating patients. An expert in clinical simulation, he teaches health assessment, evidence-based practice, and nursing education at the undergraduate and graduate levels.

Kathleen Leslie

Kathleen Leslie is an assistant professor in the Faculty of Health Disciplines at Athabasca University. She is a registered nurse and a lawyer who teaches and conducts research in various areas of health law and policy. Kate is the governance and regulation lead of the Canadian Health Workforce Network.

Sherri Melrose

Sherri Melrose facilitates undergraduate and graduate courses in the education of health professionals at Athabasca University in Alberta, Canada. She has taught a variety of theory and clinical courses, specializing in the areas of psychiatric mental health nursing and teaching and learning. Sherri has published widely on educating health professionals and is a winner of the Canadian Association of Schools of Nursing Award for Excellence in Nursing Education.

Karin Page-Cutrara

Karin Page-Cutrara, PhD RN CCNE CCSNE, is an associate professor, teaching stream at York University's School of Nursing in Toronto, Canada. Karin obtained a BNSc at Queen's University in Kingston, Ontario; a master of nursing at Athabasca University, Alberta; and a PhD in 2015 at Duquesne University, Pittsburgh, Pennsylvania, United States. She has taught as a perioperative clinical nurse educator in the hospital setting and in perioperative nursing programs as a clinical instructor in various colleges. Committed to the teaching-learning process, she uses simulation to teach clinical reasoning and clinical judgement skills to undergraduate students. Karin is a co-editor of The Role of the Nurse Educator in Canada, published in 2020 by the Canadian Association of Schools of Nursing.

Beth Perry

Beth Perry teaches undergraduate and graduate courses in the Faculty of Health Disciplines at Athabasca University, Alberta, Canada. Beth has conducted research related to exemplary nursing care, exemplary educators, and art-based inspired instruction. Beth is a past winner of the Canadian Association of Schools of Nursing Award for Excellence in Nursing Education.

Melissa Raby

Melissa Raby is the co-instructor of the Canadian Association of Schools of Nursing clinical instructor certificate course. She is a registered nurse with graduate training in public administration and public health and has held various teaching and health administration roles in both California and Ontario.

Catharine Schiller

Catharine Schiller is an assistant professor in the Faculty of Nursing at the University of Northern British Columbia. She is a registered nurse and a lawyer who teaches and conducts research into student-committed medication errors, medical assistance in dying, and nursing regulatory issues

Ruth Schofield

Ruth Schofield RN, MSc(T) is an assistant clinical professor in the Faculty of Health Sciences, School of Nursing at McMaster University. Her nursing experience of over 20 years is in public health nursing. Ruth is experienced in curriculum development, implementation, and evaluation of community health nursing education in undergraduate nursing education. She conducts research in community health nursing practice and education, and mental health and housing. Ruth is a member of the CASN Accreditation Bureau and Community Health Education Interest Group.

CHAPTER 1

Historical Context of Practice-Based Learning

Cynthia Baker

This chapter provides a historical overview of clinical placements and clinical teaching in nursing education. It describes the evolution of the clinical instructor role in the Canadian context, the diversification of clinical placements that has occurred, and the changing focus of skill development in practice-based learning.

Chapter Objectives

After completing this chapter, the reader will be able to
- outline the historical context for changes in practice-based learning in Canadian nursing education
- describe the evolving role of the clinical nursing instructor in the Canadian context
- discuss the diversification of clinical placement settings for nursing students
- describe the evolution in clinical skills fostered in nursing education

Introduction

Practice-based learning has been a critical component of nursing education in Canada since the first schools of nursing were created in the late 19th century. This chapter provides a historical overview of the changing landscape of clinical instruction in the Canadian context. In this chapter, clinical education in nursing is first situated within Canada's evolving health care system. The changing role of the clinical instructor and the diversification of clinical placements are then examined within this historical context. The chapter concludes with a discussion of the changing nature of the nursing skills fostered in practice-based learning opportunities.

Figure 1.1 Staff and First Graduating Class of the Mack Training School for Nurses

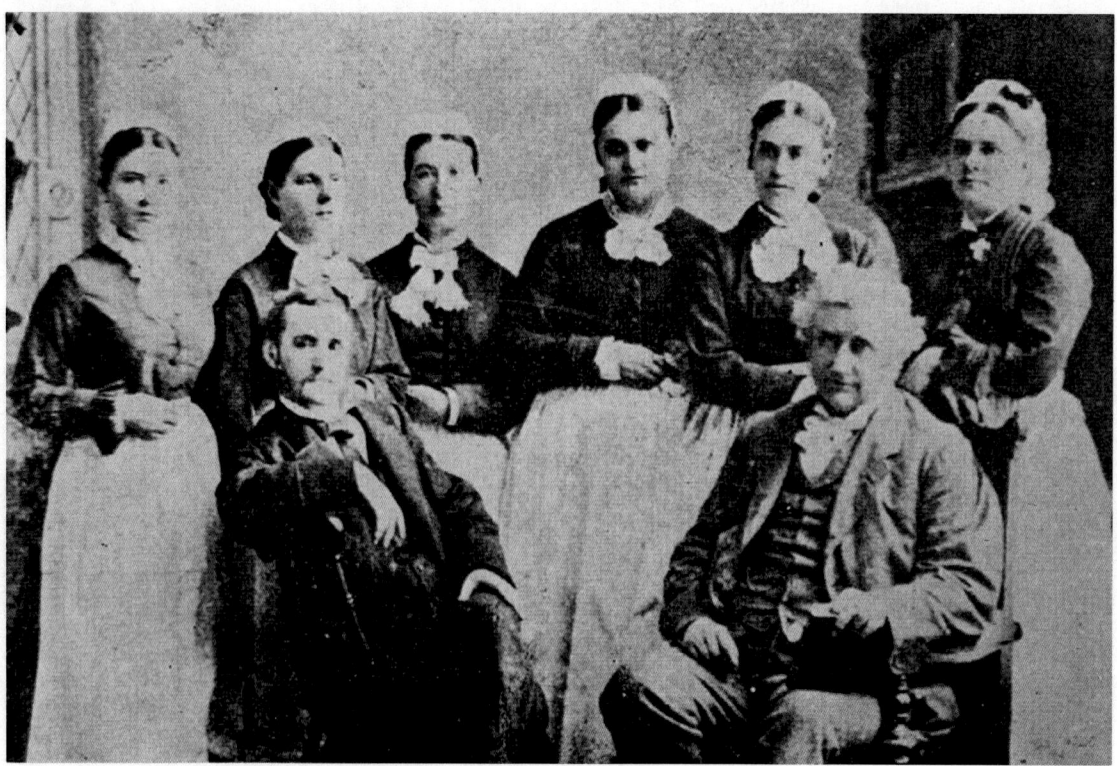

Source: From Canadian Nurse Association/Library and Archives Canada/e002414894. (n.d.). Library and Archives Canada. Item 2000-00954-9, #1. Restrictions on use: Nil. Copyright expired. https://www.bac-lac.gc.ca/eng/CollectionSearch/Pages/record.aspx?app=fonandcol&IdNumber=3604067

Overview of the Historical Background

Hospital training schools for nurses were created in the late 19th century in Canada; the first school of nursing was opened in Canada in 1874 (Figure 1.1.). Hospital training dominated nursing education in this country for almost 100 years. Following the introduction of Canada's national health care system in 1965, however, provincial and territorial jurisdictions began to move nursing education into postsecondary institutions. Despite the preponderance of hospital nursing schools, university programs for nurses were introduced in the 1920s to promote public health nursing competencies because of the 1918 flu pandemic (Duncan et al., 2020). This broadened the scope and diversity of practice-based learning in the small sector of university schools of nursing. The apprenticeship roots of nursing education, the move to postsecondary institutions, and the changing context of health care are examined in greater detail next.

Apprenticeship Roots

Formal education for nurses in Canada was introduced by Dr. Mack in St. Catharines, Ontario, with the launch of the Mack Training School for Nurses in 1874. This was the dawn of a new scientific era in medicine and the rise of hospital-based health care (Elliott et al., 2013). Inspired by Florence Nightingale, Dr. Mack believed that educated nurses would improve the outcomes for hospitalized patients and secured two Nightingale-trained instructors from England to launch the school (Canadian Association of Schools of Nursing [CASN], 2012). This model of nursing education spread rapidly as hospitals across the country began to create their own training programs for nurses.

While nursing students received some classroom courses, hospital-based training was primarily an apprenticeship. In this educational model, future practitioners of a profession or craft learn on the job. Thus, nursing students learned by doing over a three-year period in which they were assigned a progressively more demanding workload with increasing levels of responsibility, under the supervision of a charge nurse, nursing supervisor, or staff nurse during clinical rotations within the hospital (Baker, 2020).

As training schools were created to staff the burgeoning hospital system in Canada, quality issues soon emerged (Elliott et al., 2013). During this period, there were similar concerns about the apprenticeship training of physicians. Medical education, however, was completely transformed in Canada and the United States as a result of the landmark Flexner Report published in 1910. In contrast, two decades later, an evaluation of hospital training schools for nurses, sponsored by the Canadian Nurses Association and the Canadian Medical Association, had little impact. In his report published in 1932, Dr. Weir, who led the study, concluded there were significant inadequacies with hospital schools of nursing. He recommended that nursing education be removed from service and placed in universities. In contrast with the Flexner report, however, except for a few school closures, nothing changed; hospital-based training for nurses continued to flourish until well into the latter half of the 20th century.

University Education for Nurses

Despite the dominance of hospital-based training for nurses, universities in Canada introduced programs to prepare students to provide public health nursing during the 1920s in response to the 1918 flu pandemic. Typical topics in public health nursing at the time included health teaching, school health, control of communicable diseases, social work principles, and administrative and organizational principles (Duncan et al., 2020). The first baccalaureate program for nurses was launched by the University of British Columbia in 1920 and incorporated public health. Baccalaureate programs slowly increased over the next three decades, and their curricula included placements for practice-based experiences in the community and in hospitals.

Hall Commission

In 1965, the ground-breaking Hall Commission Report on health care in Canada resulted in the creation of the national health care system. It also recommended the removal of nursing education from the service sector (Baker, 2020). The goal was to have 75% of nurses educated in diploma programs and 25% in baccalaureate programs. Although most schools provided diploma-based programs, by the mid-1960s, there were already one or more baccalaureate nursing programs in most jurisdictions, and 10 new baccalaureate programs were established in response to specific recommendations in the Hall Commission Report (Baker, 2020).

With the demise of the apprenticeship model, a new approach to practice-based learning began to evolve. Because the hospital no longer ran the education program, service agreements between schools and the health care agencies were necessary to secure clinical placements. Clinical rotations were shortened considerably to allow more time for classroom-based learning, and clinical instructors (CIs) employed by the school of nursing accompanied groups of students to the service agency. These instructors were responsible for the students during their clinical placement.

Initially, many of the new diploma programs were two years. Because students provided a great deal of service in the hospital-based training program, it was assumed that they could learn what was required in considerably less time. When the first graduates joined the workforce, however, there were major concerns. Unlike the hospital-trained nurses who entered the workforce seamlessly, both diploma- and baccalaureate-prepared nurses lacked clinical skills, time management skills, and the clinical judgement to manage the full workload of a staff nurse. Kramer (1974) developed the concept of reality shock to capture what new graduates experienced in the United States on entering practice. Nursing graduates in Canada faced similar challenges (Boychuk Duchscher, 2008). As a result, many diploma programs added more practice experiences at the end of the program, and both baccalaureate and diploma programs began to introduce a final, end-of-program preceptorship.

Increasing Complexity of Health Care

At the time of the Hall Commission Report (1964, 1965), the health care system was hospital-based, and hospitals were where most nurses worked. This began to change in the decades following the report, and by 2012 only 62% of Canadian registered nurses were employed in the acute care sector (Canadian Institute for Health Information, 2012). In addition, the complexity of health care increased steadily in the decades after the Hall Commission analysis of health services. Furthermore, with the ambulatory care movement at the end of the 20th century, patient acuity in hospitals increased, length of stay shortened, and the level of nursing expertise in all sectors of health care increased exponentially (Baker, 2020). By the beginning of the 21st century, jurisdictions across Canada, except in Quebec, adopted the baccalaureate as the entry to practice in response to the increased depth and breadth of knowledge and skills nursing graduates required.

These changes added public health and community-based clinical placements to all programs for registered nurses. They also increased the challenge of providing nursing students with optimum practice-based learning experiences. The Carnegie Foundation in the United States sponsored a major study examining the demands of educating nurses for the "complex high stakes professional practice" in which "knowledge and technological innovation are increasing at an astonishing rate" (Benner et al., 2010, p. 57). The study findings emphasized the importance of skillful teaching of students in clinical placements.

Summary of the Historical Context

Practice-based learning in nursing was initially rooted in a hospital-based health care system and an apprenticeship model for practice-based learning. Clinical education and health care delivery have changed significantly in recent decades and both health care and nursing education have become more complex. These changes have impacted the role expectations of the CI, diversified placement settings, and influenced an evolution in practice skill development.

Evolution of the Clinical Instructor Role

In the hospital training schools, nurses employed by the hospital assigned tasks to students, supervised them, and evaluated their performance. When nursing education moved to postsecondary institutions, instructors employed by the educational institution accompanied students to clinical placements in hospitals and took over the staff nurses' responsibilities for students. Thus, the initial expectations for the CI role were grounded in the apprenticeship training model of the hospital schools of nursing. In recent years, however, there has been a growing emphasis on the pedagogical aspects of the CI role.

Supervisory Expectations

Service agreements between the educational institution and placement agencies often make clear that students are in clinical placements to learn, not to provide service. In hospital placements, even though staff nurses are assigned to patients being cared for by students and maintain responsibility for these patients, the CI is responsible for the students and for the care they provide. As a result, student supervision has often been understood to be the paramount expectation of CIs during hospital placements, especially supervision of students carrying out tasks (Oermann et al., 2018).

In non-clinical nursing courses, students are given time to progressively achieve the learning outcomes set for the course. With the emphasis on student supervision, CIs in hospital settings were often expected to make summative judgements about their students' performance from the beginning of the clinical placement. The need for students to have time to learn and receive adequate feedback before being evaluated was not recognized because the focus was on overseeing students' work (Oermann et al., 2018).

Indirect Supervision

The nature of community or public health nursing created a different set of role expectations for the CI. In these clinical courses, instructors do not necessarily accompany the students to the placement setting. They may work with on-site preceptors in fostering student learning, or they may guide the students on their own. In either case, much of their supervision of students' performance is indirect, although it may be supplemented with on-site observation. Meetings with students are carried out to guide their progress during the clinical placement. Thus, while the role includes supervision of students' performance, it is often at a distance, and facilitating student learning is a more central expectation.

Teaching Role

With the increasing complexity and specialization of the clinical setting, the emphasis on supervising students has been shifting. In recent years, there has been a growing emphasis on modeling ethical, professional behaviour and clinical expertise, on supporting students, and on facilitating student learning (Woodley, 2018). To promote the teaching role of CIs, for example, Oermann and colleagues (2018) developed a five-step educational process for clinical placements that actively fosters student learning. The first step is to specify learning outcomes for the clinical placement, although these are often determined by the program rather than by the CI. Students will have had different prior experiences, so the second is to assess student learning needs in relation to the learning outcomes. Learning activities are then planned to achieve the outcomes. This includes preparing for the clinical course before it begins, planning conferences during the clinical placement, selecting assignments for students, and establishing mechanisms to keep lines of communication open between students and staff. During the clinical placement, the CI guides learning through coaching, questioning, supporting, and modelling methods. The final step includes both formative and summative evaluations.

Summary of the Evolving Clinical Instructor Role

The CI role was created when nursing education moved from service agencies to educational institutions. Although it has always been recognized as a teaching role, the focus has often been on supervising students in the clinical setting. In recent years, however, facilitating learning has been given greater attention, and pedagogical approaches have been developed to foster student learning during a clinical placement. CASN has created competencies to guide CIs in their role (see Appendix).

Diversification of Practice Experiences

There has been a progressive diversification of clinical placements in the decades since nursing education moved from hospital-based training to postsecondary educational institutions. This has brought new challenges that have influenced the structure and organization of clinical education in nursing.

Increase in Placement Settings

In the hospital-based training programs, nursing students did most, if not all, their clinical rotations in the hospital that was providing the training. As noted, when nursing education moved to educational institutions, schools had to negotiate clinical placements with clinical agencies. As a result, in areas with more than one acute care hospital, nursing students began to have practice experiences in several hospitals during their program. Groups of students could also be sent to different institutions within a single clinical course.

With the evolution in health care delivery, and the baccalaureate as entry-to-practice clinical in most Canadian jurisdictions, clinical placements expanded to include multiple traditional and non-traditional settings, such as long-term-care facilities, community health centres, schools, street clinics, youth centres, Indigenous community health centres, assertive outreach programs, food banks, correctional facilities, and mental health agencies (Baker, 2020).

The variety of clinical experiences has fostered a broader and less context-based understanding of nursing practice. The diversification, however, has also brought new challenges. These include difficulties in securing appropriate placements for students and the need for new mechanisms to ensure the integrity of the curriculum across placement sites.

Increased Enrolments

The challenges resulting from the diversification of clinical placement sites have been amplified by the increase in nursing student enrolments in Canada, which have more than doubled in the last decade (CASN, 2019). This has greatly increased the number of contractually hired CIs and created the need to ensure consistency in the clinical education students receive.

Strategies developed to address potential inconsistencies include ongoing mentorship of CIs by regular faculty; well-developed resource materials, such as handbooks and reference materials; and a formal orientation to the school, the curriculum, the clinical course, and the placement site (Woodley, 2018). As both the school and the CIs must be able to work effectively with the agency staff members and build good relationships with them, the importance of CIs possessing the interpersonal skills to collaborate effectively with service agency staff has been increasingly recognized (Woodley, 2018).

Summary of the Diversification of Clinical Education

In the decades following the Hall Commission Report (1964, 1965), clinical placements became progressively more diverse. While this diversity helps students to grasp general nursing principles and differentiate these from context-specific expectations, it has increased the organizational demands of clinical education and requires new mechanisms to promote greater consistency in the clinical education that instructors provide students.

Clinical Skill Development

Overall, the purpose of clinical placements is to provide nursing students with practice experiences that foster the development of the competencies they will need on entering the health care workforce. Although students must possess a set of cognitive, affective, relational, and psychomotor skills and abilities to manifest a given competency (Tardiff, 2006), it was often the student's ability to perform tasks that was prioritized in clinical settings. An increasing emphasis on the development of relational skills in clinical education, however, was evident at the end of the 20th century, and in recent years, cognitive skill development has been a focus.

Task Orientation

In hospital-based training programs, students rotated from one unit to another for varying periods of time. At the beginning of their program, they carried out simpler tasks, and as they gained experience, assumed more complex ones. Although hospitals moved from distributing tasks among the nursing staff and students to assigning patients to nurses, an emphasis on task performance continued. At the beginning of their program, students cared for fewer patients and were assigned patients with less complex needs. Their workload increased progressively, and by the third year, students were often expected to carry a full patient assignment and all responsibilities of a staff nurse (Baker, 2020).

Students' abilities to work quickly, efficiently, and correctly were highly valued and emerged through practice, as did their ability to prioritize when facing competing demands on their time. On graduating from the program, their entry into the workforce was seamless. However, health care services and the nursing role were far simpler then than they are today.

The focus on students' ability to carry out tasks appropriately persisted for decades in clinical placements, as did the expectation that new graduates should be able to begin a full workload immediately. As early as the 1950s and 1960s, however, nursing scholars began to stress the need for students to develop a broader skill set in clinical placements, including relational abilities and cognitive skills.

Relational Skills

In 1952, Hildegarde Peplau published a theory of interpersonal relations in which she described nursing as an interpersonal process and identified the nurse-patient relationship as the foundation of nursing practice. In her theory, the nurse uses the "self" therapeutically. She identified the following phases of a therapeutic nurse-patient relationship: orientation, working, and termination (Peplau, 1952).

Less than 15 years later, Joyce Travelbee (1966) published *Interpersonal Aspects of Nursing*. Influenced by existentialism, Travelbee envisioned nursing as an interpersonal process aimed at helping individuals and their families to prevent or manage illness and suffering. She understood sympathy as going beyond empathy, with nurses actively seeking to lessen the suffering experienced by patients and supporting them in finding meaning in suffering (Travelbee, 1966).

The early emphasis on relational skills advanced by Peplau and Travelbee grew in the late 1980s and throughout the 1990s because of the work of Jean Watson. In 1979, Watson published the *Philosophy and Science of Caring* and in 1985, *Human Science and Human Care – A Theory of Nursing*. In her model, caring is identified as the essence of nursing (Watson, 1979). Several Canadian schools of nursing specifically adopted Watson's model of nursing to guide their curricula, and increased attention was paid in nursing education to caring relationships in clinical placements.

More recently, Doane and Varcoe (2015) developed the concept of relational inquiry, which has had an important impact on clinical instruction in Canada. In this approach, the broader social context in which clients and their support systems are situated is critical. Nurses' awareness of themselves and how they influence and are connected to the client and the health care system is also central. Nursing students are encouraged to adopt the perspective of an inquirer and to enact an inquiry process. As inquirers, nurses enter each nursing situation by inquiring into the relational experience of people, including themselves, and into contexts, knowledge, meaningful purposes, excellence of practices, and effectiveness of outcomes (Doane & Varcoe, 2015).

Cognitive Skills

Recently, emphasis on fostering the development of cognitive processes to guide nursing action has been growing (Oermann et al., 2018). Several overlapping concepts have been used to describe the cognitive abilities students should develop in clinical placements, including problem solving, critical thinking, sense of salience, clinical reasoning, and clinical judgement.

Problem Solving

Despite the longstanding focus on tasks, nursing scholars began developing cognitive approaches to guide nursing in the 1950s and 1960s. Orlando (1961) argued that nursing actions must be undertaken deliberately based on a problem-solving nursing process. This process includes identifying and defining a nursing problem, collecting data related to the problem, proposing and implementing solutions, and evaluating the outcome (Oermann et al.,

2018). This process continues to be used in nursing practice and education, but often the problems identified, and the interventions selected, are drawn from a standardized list.

Critical Thinking

Critical thinking is also being promoted in clinical courses. Multiple definitions of the concept exist, however, and it is often used interchangeably with problem solving or as a catch-all generic phrase to capture the complex thinking nurses use in practice (Benner et al., 2010). Elements of critical thinking to be fostered in clinical placements include having a questioning attitude, not taking information at face value, considering alternative perspectives and explanations, seeking answers, and being open-minded (Oermann et al., 2018).

Sense of Salience

Because nurses face multiple competing demands among their assigned clients, which change as patient care situations evolve, a common safety concern is that new nursing graduates are unable to determine what is most important to respond to at a given time. Benner and colleagues introduced the notion of a *sense of salience* to capture a key cognitive process needed for this. The concept refers to the nurse's ability to evaluate situations as a whole and to determine what are most and least important (Benner et al., 2010).

CIs are encouraged to ask students skillful questions to foster the development of an initial sense of salience. The aim is to facilitate the student's awareness that although most patient care goals are important, they are not equally urgent, as well as to create an awareness that priorities may need to be revised as a clinical situation evolves (Benner et al., 2010).

Clinical Reasoning

The need for nursing students to develop clinical reasoning skills is receiving increasing attention in clinical teaching. It is commonly understood to be a cognitive process of making sense of a clinical situation as it unfolds (Cappelletti et al., 2014). Like problem solving, clinical reasoning includes observing, collecting, and analyzing patient information; evaluating the significance of these data; and weighing alternative actions (Simmons, 2010). In contrast, however, clinical reasoning is characterized by recursive metacognition and cognitive processes (Deschênes & Goudreau, 2017). Distinguishing characteristics of clinical reasoning that are being fostered in clinical courses include encouraging students to generate hypotheses to interpret dynamic and often ambiguous clinical situations and to weigh alternative actions.

Clinical Judgement

Although definitions of clinical judgement focus on coming to a conclusion about a patient's needs or concerns and determining what action, if any, to take, models of clinical judgement tend to go beyond the definition of the concept. Some incorporate the clinical reasoning processes that precede the interpretations of observations and information; others include both the clinical reasoning processes and a cognitive reflection process on the action taken; and, finally, some also include the implementation of the nursing action itself, as well as clinical reasoning processes that occur before the clinical judgement and the reflections that occur after the nursing action is taken (Baker, 2020).

The Tanner model has been an influential conceptualization of clinical judgement, albeit one that goes beyond arriving at an interpretation or conclusion (Tanner, 2006). It includes a four-stage cognitive process initiated by a perceptual grasp of a situation that is not necessarily the outcome of an assessment (noticing). Interpreting the situation follows and leads to a course of action (responding). The final stage involves reflecting while responding and then reflecting on the results (Tanner, 2006).

Pedagogical strategies to develop clinical judgement in clinical placements include coaching students to notice deviations from expected patterns, encouraging them to deliberately seek out information about their observation, and using questions to encourage students to analyze observations, to prioritize, and to reflect on clinical actions taken. Often, students are prepared during pre-conferences to be aware of these cognitive stages and are guided in reflecting on actions taken during post-conference discussions.

Summary of Clinical Skill Development

As nursing education was grounded in an apprenticeship model, there was a focus on the tasks to be performed by students in clinical placements, which persisted for many years despite a move to holistic models of nursing care. A strong emphasis, however, on fostering student's relational engagement with clients and the social determinants affecting their health has been evident in clinical courses since the last decade of the 20th century. In addition, in recent years, the increasing complexity, ambiguity, and fluidity of clinical situations have strengthened the attention given to cognitive skill development to guide caregiving in dynamic and changing contexts.

Summary of the Chapter

Education for nurses in Canada was introduced in the late 19th century, inspired by Florence Nightingale's understanding of the profession. The early schools, however, were not the independent institutions envisioned by Nightingale, and nursing students soon became a major component of the hospital workforce. The movement of nursing education to postsecondary institutions changed the organization and delivery of practice-based learning. The CI role has evolved from supervisor to educator; the number and type of clinical placement sites for students have multiplied; and while task development skills continue to be important, increasing attention has been given to fostering relational skills and cognitive skill development in practice-based learning activities.

Conclusion

The health care system, nursing roles, and nursing competencies have evolved significantly since the first school of nursing was opened in Canada in 1874. Practice-based learning, however, was, and continues to be, an integral component of nursing education. Currently, schools of nursing are charged with preparing students to enter a highly complex and specialized profession successfully. As the historical context of practice-based learning indicates, the CI role and clinical placement experiences are essential in achieving this goal.

References

Baker, C. (2020). Clinical nursing education in the Canadian context. In K. Page-Cutrara & P. Bradley (Eds.), *The role of the nurse educator in Canada* (pp. 220–237). Canadian Association of Schools of Nursing.

Benner, P., Sutphen, M., Leonard, V., & Day, L. (2010). *Educating nurses. A call for radical transformation*. Jossey-Bass; Carnegie Foundation for the Advancement of Teaching.

Boychuk Duchscher, J. (2008). A process of becoming: The stages of new nursing graduates' professional role transition. *The Journal of Continuing Education in Nursing, 39*(10), 441–450. https://doi.org/10.3928/00220124-20081001-03

Canadian Association of Schools of Nursing. (2012). *Ties that bind: The evolution of education for professional nursing in Canada from the 17th century to the 21st century*.

Canadian Institute for Health Information. (2012). *Regulated nurses: Canadian trends, 2007 to 2011*.

Cappelletti, A., Engel, J., & Prentice, D. (2014). Systematic review of clinical judgement and reasoning in nursing. *Journal of Nursing Education, 62*(8), 453–458. https://doi.org/10.3928/01484834-20140724-01

Deschênes, M.-F., & Goudreau, J. (2017). Addressing the development of both knowledge and clinical reasoning in nursing through the perspective of script concordance: An integrative review. *Journal of Nursing Education & Practice, 7*(12), 28. https://doi.org/10.5430/jnep.v7n12p28

Doane, H. G., & Varcoe, C. (2015). *How to nurse? Relational inquiry with individuals and families in changing health and healthcare contexts*. Williams & Wilkins.

Duncan, S., Scala, M., & Boschma, G. (2020). 100 Years of university nursing education: Its origins and significance for nursing now. *Quality Advancement in Nursing Education – Avancées en formation infirmière, 6*(2). https://qane-afi.casn.ca/journal/vol6/iss2/8

Elliott, J., Rutty, C., & Villeneuve, M. (2013). *One hundred years of service, 1908-2008*. Canadian Nurses Association.

Flexner, A. (1910). *Medical education in the United States and Canada: A report to the Carnegie Foundation for the Advancement of Teaching*. Carnegie Foundation for the Advancement of Teaching. http://archive.carnegiefoundation.org/publications/pdfs/elibrary/Carnegie_Flexner_Report.pdf

Hall, E. (1964). *Royal commission on health services, 1964: Volume 1*. Privy Council Office. https://publications.gc.ca/site/eng/9.818794/publication.html

Hall, E. (1965). *Royal commission on health services, 1964: Volume 2*. Privy Council Office. https://publications.gc.ca/site/eng/9.818827/publication.html

Kramer, M. (1974). *Reality shock: Why nurses leave nursing*. Mosby.

Oermann, M. H., Shellenbarger, T., & Gaberson, K. B. (2018). *Clinical teaching strategies in nursing* (5th ed.). Springer.

Orlando, I. J. (1961). *The dynamic nurse patient relationship. Function, process and principles*. G.P. Putman.

Peplau, H. (1952). *Interpersonal relations in nursing: A conceptual frame of reference for psychodynamic nursing*. G.P. Putnam.

Simmons, B. (2010). Clinical reasoning: Concept analysis. *Journal of Advanced Nursing, 66*, 1151–1558. https://doi.org/10.1111/j.1365-2648.2010.05262x

Tanner, C. (2006). Thinking like a nurse: A research-based model of clinical judgement in nursing. *Journal of Nursing Education, 45*(6), 204–211. https://doi.org/10.3928/01484834-20060601-04

Tardiff, J. (2006). *L'evaluation des compétences. Documenter le parcours de d'eveloppement*. Chenelière Education.

Travelbee, J. (1966). *Interpersonal aspects of nursing*. F.A. Davis.

Watson, J. (1979). *Nursing: The philosophy and science of caring*. University Press of Colorado.

Watson, J. (1985). *Nursing: Human science and human care: a theory of nursing*. Appleton-Century-Crofts.

Weir, G. (1932). *Survey of nursing education in Canada*. University of Toronto Press.

Woodley, L. (2018). Clinical teaching in nursing. In M. J. Oermann, J. C. De Gagne, & B. Cusatis Philips (Eds.), *Teaching in nursing and role of the educator* (pp. 179–202). Springer.

CHAPTER 2

The Role of the Clinical Instructor

Sherri Melrose

This chapter examines the role of the clinical instructor in Canada. Characteristics of an effective educator are discussed, elements of curricula are outlined, and successful collaborations are considered.

Chapter Objectives

After completing this chapter, the reader will be able to
- discuss the characteristics of an effective educator
- outline the elements of program and course curricula
- describe how to establish successful collaborations

Introduction

Nursing is a practice-based profession, and clinical learning experiences play an important role in helping student nurses to develop the knowledge, skills, and attitudes they need to work in a wide range of practice settings and specialty areas. The role of the clinical instructor (CI) is to facilitate students' progress and to prepare them to meet entry-to-practice competencies.

To fulfil that role, CIs must extend their expertise as practitioners to also become effective educators. They must demonstrate a comprehensive understanding of the curriculum their students are required to follow at both the program and the course level. They must also understand the policies, procedures, and everyday tasks in the clinical areas where they teach students. As key members of both academic communities and practice communities, CIs are required to establish collaborations among their students, their faculty colleagues, and the health professionals they encounter in clinical placements. To help define this role, CASN created a set of competencies for the CI (see Appendix).

Straddling the complexities of the CI role is not easy. This chapter presents a broad overview of what novice nurses can be expected to know when they take on the role of CI. Following a brief discussion of the background and history of the CI role in Canada, a general discussion of the characteristics of effective educators is presented. Basic elements essential to understanding program and course curricula are outlined. Considerations for establishing successful collaborations are described. Throughout the chapter, emphasis is placed on the positive impact an educator's own commitment to lifelong learning can have on the CI role.

Background and History of Clinical Instructor Role in Canada

As Chapter 1 explains, practice-based learning in Canada has changed significantly over the years. Registered nurses (RNs) were not always educated in universities. Traditionally, they acquired skills by providing services or unpaid work to organizations in return for an education. Known as *service for training*, this approach to learning was grounded in an apprenticeship model, where, as the name implies, training was provided in return for service (Canadian Association of Schools of Nursing [CASN], 2012; Wytenbroek & Vandenberg, 2017).

In addition to attending classes, students were instructed and supervised by senior nurses in the workplace. Student nurses worked alongside practising nurses and were expected to function as contributing members of patient care teams. Although these practising nurses were not identified as CIs, they were among the first to undertake this role.

Before the 1990s, most schools of nursing were housed in hospitals, and hospitals relied heavily on student nurses to provide care for patients. Therefore, students' clinical education often revolved around hospital workplace requirements, and hospital administrators controlled many educational practices (Melrose et al., 2020). Classrooms were often located right on the hospital units and the role of the instructor included teaching in both classroom and clinical areas.

It was not until hospital schools of nursing moved into community colleges and university settings that the role of an educator dedicated exclusively to clinical instruction was identified. By 2000, Canadian RNs were required to hold a baccalaureate degree in nursing (Pringle et al., 2004). The transition away from hospital-based training programs granting diplomas and towards university-based programs granting baccalaureate degrees led to more specialized educational roles.

With classrooms situated in university buildings, travel to hospitals and other clinical placement areas was cumbersome. Faculty employed at universities were expected to lead and implement research projects, leaving less time for clinical teaching. In turn, the shifting demands of the academic role created opportunities for expert clinicians to step in as CIs and share their hands-on knowledge and skills with student nurses. Thus, the role of CI is still relatively new, and the associated responsibilities and expectations continue to evolve.

However, the CI role is clearly an educational role that requires demonstration of effective instruction. The next section discusses how expertise, positive role modelling, and a passion for the profession are characteristics of effective educators that are especially relevant to clinical instruction.

Characteristics of Effective Educators

Expertise

Effective educators bring expertise to their role. For CIs, this expertise includes clinical knowledge and instructional knowledge. CIs are expert practitioners, making the skills and experiences they share with students highly valued. Additionally, CIs expertise must also include instructional knowledge. Fostering and maintaining clinical and instructional expertise is an inherent expectation of all nurses who take on the CI role.

Clinical Expertise

To be effective educators, CIs must have the content knowledge associated with their area of expertise (Collier, 2018; Niederriter et al., 2017; Reising et al., 2018; Sadeghi et al., 2019). Before educators can help students transfer knowledge from lectures, labs, simulations, and other program learning activities to the clinical setting, they must first have a comprehensive understanding of the subject matter themselves.

When CIs' maintain their clinical competence, they project confidence (Niederriter et al., 2017; Reising et al., 2018). In turn, CIs who feel confident in their own practice inspire similar feelings of confidence in their students, thereby creating more meaningful learning experiences (Collier, 2018; Needham et al., 2016; Niederriter et al., 2017; Reising et al., 2018; Sadeghi et al., 2019). Conversely, CIs who lack current clinical knowledge and who are unfamiliar with common procedures in their clinical area hinder the quality of students' experiences (Reising et al., 2018).

When accepting an offer of employment as a new CI, nurses must assess their capacity to practise competently in a particular clinical area. This assessment includes considering the applicability of their existing experience and available professional development opportunities. Schools of nursing may provide compensation for time spent orienting to a clinical teaching area, but CIs are responsible for identifying their own learning needs and finding the resources to meet these needs. Examples include attending national and international conferences focused on clinical topics, reviewing literature related to conditions commonly occurring in the area, attending staff in-services, buddying with staff, and practising with equipment that students will use. Although educators can never prepare for all contingencies, initiating self-directed learning strategies well in advance of meeting students establishes a strong foundation.

Instructional Expertise

CIs are educators, yet the responsibilities inherent in an educator role can be overshadowed by the pressures of maintaining clinical competence. Instructional competence requires CIs to seek out information and tools from the discipline of education that will allow them to convey their knowledge and teach others. In many instances, undergraduate and graduate programs have not provided nurses with this foundation to being an excellent teacher. Therefore, once again, CIs must be self-directed and look for opportunities to strengthen their knowledge of teaching and learning. Chapter 3 introduces readers to the pedagogy of clinical teaching.

Opportunities for developing instructional competence include completing continuing education courses such as those offered by the CASN's Canadian Nurse Educator Institute (2022). Similarly, graduate studies courses focused on teaching and learning are available to non-program students in the Faculty of Health Disciplines at Athabasca University, Canada's online university (Athabasca University, n.d.). Informally, CIs can read refereed journals, books, and open educational resources (OER) geared to nurse educators. OERs are free online resources that can be accessed anytime and anywhere. One example of an OER of value to Canadian CIs is *Creative Clinical Teaching in the Health Professions* (Melrose et al., 2021).

CIs who cultivate and demonstrate their instructional expertise have a positive impact on students' learning (Needham et al., 2016; Niederriter et al., 2017; Sweet & Broadbent, 2017). Conveying knowledge to others involves a different skill set than acquiring knowledge, and students appreciate CIs who know how to pass along what they know (Janse van Rensburg, 2019; Reising et al., 2018). When CIs are unable to convey their knowledge effectively, students perceive them as disorganized, inefficient, and out of their depth (Needham et al., 2016).

Positive Role Modelling

Effective educators are positive role models. A role model is a person worthy of emulation, a positive example of a member of the profession (Perry, 2009). Students see behaviours that they aspire to and want to emulate in all their educators, but in clinical settings, CIs can and should model the kinds of professional behaviours they expect from students. Students pattern their own actions on what they see CIs doing during their everyday interactions and activities, as well as when they are providing formal instruction. Whether intentionally or unintentionally, what CIs *do* can exert more influence than what they *say* (Melrose et al., 2020).

When students observe CIs consistently role modelling positivity, enthusiasm, and caring, they feel more satisfied with their learning experiences (Jack et al., 2017). CIs can consciously integrate positive role modelling behaviours by communicating a supportive attitude, an approachable demeanor, and a passion for the profession.

Supportive Attitude

Students need to feel unwavering support from their CIs. They must trust that CIs will always be there for them as a guide and an advocate (Niederriter et al., 2017). Wanting to thrive in clinical settings, students rely on CIs to help them find ways to reduce anxiety, to understand what is expected of them, and to achieve required competencies. CIs can begin to communicate a supportive attitude by acknowledging and normalizing feelings of anxiety, by projecting a willingness to remain emotionally available, and by displaying patience (Janse van Rensburg, 2019).

It is common for students to use the same verbal and non-verbal expressions of support with their patients that they experienced during interactions with their CIs. In some instances, students even replicate CIs mannerisms and colloquial language. This observation serves as a reminder to CIs that the interactions they are modelling with (and in front of) students can have a profound and lasting impact.

Approachable Demeanour

When CIs present an approachable demeanour to students, they invite conversations and questions that might not otherwise emerge. Students are more able to accept feedback (both positive and constructive) from CIs who are approachable. An approachable CI is friendly, respectful, and generally relaxed, and readily establishes relationships with most members of health care teams (Collier, 2018; Hababeh & Lalithabai, 2020; Niederriter et al., 2017; Reising et al., 2018; Sweet & Broadbent, 2017).

Approachability can be communicated through simple gestures such as smiling frequently, making eye contact, stopping a task whenever possible to talk, and expressing genuine interest in students' comments and questions. During times of crisis in clinical settings, these expressions of approachability can easily be neglected. CIs inadvertently may use a brusque tone or utter a sharp word. In these instances, acknowledging and apologizing for lapses that have occurred can also communicate approachability. Here again, CIs are modelling behaviour they expect from students, who will also have times where they appear unapproachable to others.

Knowing that CIs evaluate their progress, students can feel hesitant to reach out for help. Fearing reprisal, students may be reluctant to disclose errors, and that fear results in unsafe patient care. Overcoming the inherent power differential in instructor-student relationships is not easy. Yet when CIs make a conscious effort to communicate that they are willing to be approached, students are more likely to feel safe in doing so.

For many students, approaching a CI is viewed as a risk. Negative experiences with previous educators, lack of success in other educational activities, cultural barriers, traumatic life experiences, and other personal factors can all influence students' decisions to approach (or not approach) CIs.

CIs who identify how to reach them communicate that they are approachable. Throughout each clinical shift, students must know the specific times and communication devices to use to connect with their CI. In traditional clinical settings, such as hospitals or clinics, where instructors and students remain in the same building, CIs may expect students to come and find them. In clinical settings where CIs travel between sites, communication may occur through telephone, text, email, or online learning platforms. When CIs facilitate clinical learning online, they may use additional social media tools.

It is important for newly employed CIs to understand the expected methods of communication between students and CIs. For example, some nursing programs may encourage CIs to implement communication tools commonly used by the public. Others may impose restrictions on their use. Additionally, CIs must consider their own personal boundaries and let students know the times they are not available.

Passion for the Profession

Enthusiastic, positive CIs who love what they do and who feel excited about sharing their knowledge with the next generation of nurses are strong role models. Students appreciate knowing why their educators chose the nursing profession, what areas sparked (and continue to spark) their interest, and how they find joy in their work. CIs communicate their passion for teaching by genuinely valuing students' successes and taking pride in students' accomplishments.

On the other hand, when CIs seem to focus on what is not going well, challenges not being overcome, and barriers being imposed by programs or clinical sites, any feelings of passion they may have for the profession are muffled. Students view this apparent lack of passion as apathy and even laziness (Reising et al., 2018). When CIs seem more interested in focusing on mistakes than successes, they are viewed as dispassionate, intimidating, and condescending (Reising et al., 2018).

In addition to embodying the characteristics of effective educators described above, the CI role requires a basic understanding of the program and course curricula of the schools of nursing in which the CIs are employed. These elements are outlined next.

Elements of Program and Course Curricula

CIs are required to have a general understanding of the curricula that guide students' programs and a more in-depth grasp of the curriculum for the specific clinical course they are teaching. The term *curricula* refers to different educational and instructional practices. A *curriculum,* the singular form of curricula, is defined as a formal plan of study that provides the philosophical underpinnings, goals, and guidelines for delivery and evaluation methods that a specific educational program will implement (Keating, 2015; Melrose et al., 2020).

The word derives from the Latin *currere*, which carried directly over into English and means "running a race [or a] course," with a secondary meaning of running around a racetrack (Egan, 1978, p. 10). The metaphor of running a race suggests that curricula, like racetracks, have predetermined structures clearly in place. Curricular structures include explicit plans for learners to interact with instructional content and processes and for evaluating the attainment of educational goals (Melrose et al., 2020).

Program Curricula

At the program level, CIs can begin to understand curricula by reviewing the program's website. Program websites are a key source of information for prospective and current nursing students, and they can be a valuable resource for CIs as well. Reading the program philosophy, messages from leaders, courses that are required, and general directions to students will reveal important insights. Scanning course outlines will offer a snapshot of the kinds of teaching approaches, learning activities, and evaluation methods that students are familiar with. In some instances, CIs may be able to audit students' classes when topics of interest are presented.

Similarly, CIs can learn more about the program curricula that guides their students' learning by attending faculty meetings and participating in academic projects. Informal conversations with other members of the faculty group can be valuable. As attendance is voluntary, and CIs are not usually compensated, this strategy can be difficult. Because of time constraints, orientation workshops cannot provide new CIs with a total overview of all aspects of the program. These orientation sessions usually focus on the clinical courses that attendees will be teaching. Therefore, piecing together other elements of the curriculum is an individual CI responsibility.

Course Curricula

CIs can expect to be provided with curricular materials for the courses they have been hired to teach. These materials should include course guides that specify competencies that students must achieve and evaluation tools for measuring students' progress. The materials should also include relevant policies and procedures associated with the academic institution.

It is important to note that curricula are revised frequently. This is in response to the constant changes that occur in both academic and clinical environments. Consequently, CIs may receive information only as courses begin. This leaves limited time for careful review and reflection. Knowing in advance that blocks of time will be needed to review and reflect on curricular materials, CIs can adjust their schedules accordingly. The first week of a clinical course can be hectic. Experienced educators often advise new CIs to keep other work, family, and study commitments to a minimum whenever possible during this time.

Orientations to individual clinical sites are not typically included in curricular materials. Creating site orientations for students and setting up recording systems to chronicle student progress are part of the preparatory planning CIs must do on their own (Baker, 2020). Similarly, CIs must also seek out relevant policies and procedures issued by the clinical institutions.

Some documents and resources may be available on institutional websites. As access can be restricted to staff members, CIs not employed in the clinical areas where they teach students will need to apply to gain access. A strategy CIs may find helpful in organizing their student orientation package is to create a private website or use a learning management system accessible only to students currently attending a clinical site. In essence, CIs are responsible for curating information from clinical sites and finding ways to communicate this information to students.

As the above discussions illustrated, the CI role is multifaceted. At times, responsibilities associated with being an effective educator and delivering both academic and clinical curricula can feel overwhelming. Networking and creating connections with colleagues can make an important difference in ameliorating some of these feelings. Next, suggestions for establishing successful collaborations are offered.

Establishing Successful Collaborations

Instructor-Student Collaborations

Nurses who succeed in the role of CI establish successful collaborations. In their collaborative relationships with students, CIs work as supportive partners. The goal of any instructor-student partnership is to support students in achieving required course competencies. Certainly, the goal cannot be attained by instructors and students working alone. However, as emphasized throughout this book, the collaborative relationships CIs establish with students set the stage for all subsequent collaborations with other educational partners.

In genuinely collaborative instructor-student relationships, students are invited to actively engage in their learning. This includes working together to match teaching styles to learning needs (as discussed in Chapter 3) and to create safe spaces for critical reflection. This approach is built on a foundation of mutual trust and respect. CIs generate building blocks for this important foundation when they get to know students as individuals. Questions such as why students chose nursing, what area they hope to practice in, and how they handle life challenges can initiate meaningful conversations.

Successful instructor-student collaborations can only be maintained when CIs consistently remain open to the *exchange of feedback*. Collaborative feedback involves CIs providing students with feedback on their progress (instructional feedback), and it requires CIs to invite feedback on their own teaching (student feedback). In clinical settings, instructional feedback is usually based on direct observation. Students are most receptive to feedback when it is shared as soon as possible after an activity has been observed.

When students sense that their CIs are genuinely committed to supporting them to be successful rather than finding fault, their anxiety decreases. Comments should always include a balance of both positive and constructive or corrective statements and should clearly relate to course learning outcomes. Effective feedback "provide[s] an unbiased critique of performance, recounting events as they occurred, with the intention to correct errors and increase understanding" (Atmiller, 2016, p. 118). Discussions must never occur in front of other students, staff, or patients.

Similarly, any exchanges in which students share feedback on CIs activities should also be grounded in a mutual commitment to student success. Program curricula may establish only limited opportunities for students to evaluate CIs. For example, anonymous written end-of-term course evaluations may include sections where students can comment on their CI's teaching effectiveness.

Rather than waiting until the clinical experience is over, when CIs invite student feedback throughout the course, they model a process of receiving, accepting (or rejecting with explanation), and acting on feedback. Student feedback can be solicited during impromptu discussions and can be scheduled into student evaluation meetings. Student input can also be gathered anonymously in suggestion box collection areas or through online opportunities. Importantly, students must feel that their feedback is welcome and that their relationship with their CI is a collaboration.

Student-Student Collaborations

Facilitating student-student collaborations is equally important. Peer interactions, both during and outside time in clinical areas, will foster learning. Assigning student partnerships at the beginning of a rotation and then later inviting students to form their own collaborations promotes inclusivity. Providing pre- and post-clinical discussions on online platforms supported by the nursing program provides opportunities for students to share and extend their thinking with like-minded others. Requiring students to establish what they expect from one another during a collaboration (and the consequences if expectations are not met) is a facilitation strategy that CIs can implement (Melrose et al., 2013).

Successful student-student collaborations do not just happen. They must be carefully cultivated. Whether students come together in pairs or triads for activities such as skills demonstrations, in groups of three or four to complete a project assignment, or in small groups of ten or more for clinical conferences, dynamics related to group processes will occur. Understanding how groups progress and how to promote positive group dynamics is an important function of the CI role.

Most nurses are familiar with general background information on group dynamics. For example, Tuckman (1965) and Tuckman and Jensen (1977) identified that groups progress through four stages. Groups form (members learn about one another), they storm (conflicts are likely to occur), they norm and perform (they work effectively together towards a common goal), and they adjourn (close or end the group). The stages, represented in Figure 2.1, may not occur sequentially and not all groups are able to work together successfully.

Knowing that issues (such as conflict) are expected to emerge when students collaborate in groups, CIs can build in strategies to help. For example, when student partnerships and groups are first forming, they value knowing that they are not on their own, that their CIs are available if students need them, and that it's safe to contact their CI (Melrose & Bergeron, 2007; Melrose et al., 2013). When storming occurs and students struggle to manage conflict, particularly in relation to participation and evaluation, they need to be certain that their CI is willing and able to step in and help.

As students move through norming and performing, CIs can mistakenly assume that they are not needed. Although joining student groups and participating directly in discussions during this stage may not be necessary, it is important for CIs to maintain communication with all students individually. This one-to-one communication assures students that their personal learning needs and goals have not been forgotten. Finally, intentionally planning opportunities to debrief and reflect when groups adjourn provides students with closure.

Figure 2.1 *Tuckman and Jensen's (1977) Stages of Group Development*

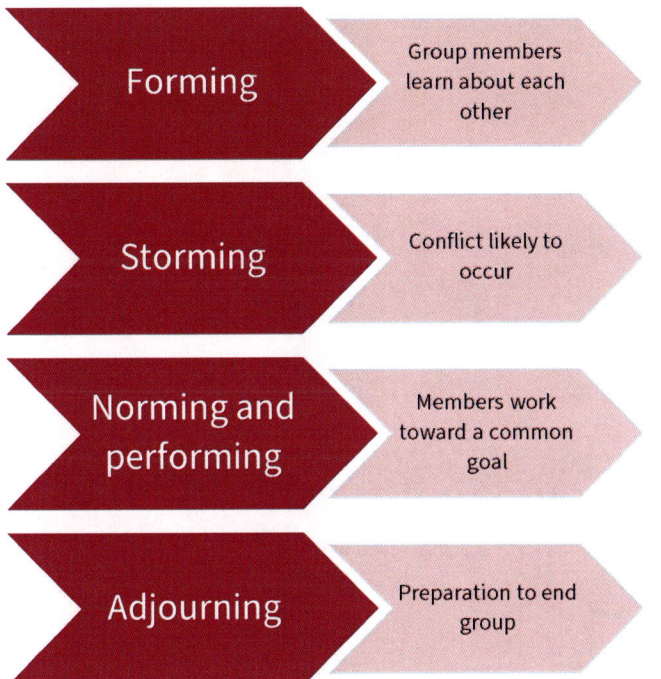

Source: Adapted from *Open Textbooks of Hong Kong* (n.d.).

Instructor-Faculty Collaborations

CIs are also required to establish successful collaborations with other faculty and instructors at the academic institution where they are employed. Although CIs may attend formal meetings only infrequently to understand program and course curricula fully, networking with colleagues can offer valuable insights. Exchanging contact information and connecting with fellow educators can quickly clear up misconceptions that may have developed. Informally sharing practical tips for navigating instructional requirements over a cup of coffee or tea can inspire new ways of thinking.

Instructor-Program Collaborations

Collaborations with nursing programs also require CIs to understand services that are available to students. For example, students may require language support services, counselling services, math tutoring, or English writing support (Melrose et al., 2020). CIs must be aware of policies associated with failing grades and grade appeals. They must know what steps both students and instructors can take if they believe they have been treated unfairly.

Notably, CIs must know well in advance the procedures to follow if they are ill or otherwise unable to attend the clinical area (Melrose et al., 2021). Unlike K–12 educational institutions, schools of nursing do not usually have lists of qualified substitute teachers who can step in and supervise students on short notice. When they are ill, CIs are required to notify all their students, the academic institution, and the clinical site in a timely manner.

Having a student contact plan in place is essential and especially useful when illness occurs just hours before a scheduled shift. Students' clinical experiences will likely be cancelled when a CI is ill. Unfortunately, clinical experiences cannot be rescheduled; shifts at the clinical placement locations are booked months, or even years, in advance, and the sites provide practical learning opportunities to learners from a variety of health profession programs. Students often travel long distances and juggle complicated childcare and employment commitments to get to clinical sites. To arrive and find their clinical experience cancelled is frustrating.

Instructor-Clinical Collaborations

Successful collaborations with administrators and staff in clinical areas are invaluable as CIs prepare nursing students for entry into the profession. Just as both formal and informal connections with academic institutions contribute to students' success, collaborations in clinical settings also make a difference. Discovering where to access policies, procedures, and resources takes time. Often, orientation programs are provided to new staff members, and when possible, attending these orientations can be useful. Instructors who taught in the area previously may have materials and information a new CI can use. For CIs not employed at the site where they teach, working alongside staff, participating in unit projects, and communicating a willingness to pitch in fosters relationships. When students' written assignments are relevant to patient care, sharing these with staff may be appreciated.

Summary

The role of the CI emerged when nursing education moved away from hospital-based service-for-training approaches to educating nurses in university settings. CIs supervise students' progress in clinical settings and prepare them to meet entry-to-practice competencies. As educators, CIs must maintain both clinical and instructional expertise. They must strive to demonstrate characteristics of effective educators, which include role modelling behaviours they expect students to emulate, communicating a supportive attitude, projecting an approachable demeanour, and sharing their passion for the nursing profession. CIs must understand elements of program and course curricula that apply to their students. Further, they are expected to establish successful collaborations with and among students and with colleagues in both the academic and the clinical institutions where they teach.

Conclusion

CIs are essential members of nursing education teams. They play a vital part in supporting students in successfully meeting learning outcomes. The CI role provides nurses with a variety of opportunities to grow as clinicians and instructors, and it creates exciting possibilities for collaborations among diverse groups of colleagues. CIs are self-directed lifelong learners who enjoy sharing what they know with future Canadian nurses.

References

Athabasca University. (n.d.). *Faculty of health disciplines.* https://fhd.athabascau.ca

Atmiller, G. (2016). Strategies for providing constructive feedback to students. *Nurse Educator, 41*(3), 118–119. https://doi.org/10.1097/NNE.0000000000000227

Baker, C. (2020). Clinical nursing education in the Canadian context. In K. Page-Cutrara & P. Bradley (Eds.), *The role of the nurse educator in Canada* (pp. 220–237). Canadian Association of Schools of Nursing.

Canadian Association of Schools of Nursing. (2012). *Ties that bind: The evolution of education for professional nursing in Canada from the 17th to the 21st century.*

Canadian Nurse Educator Institute. (2022). *Programs and courses.* http://cnei-icie.casn.ca/our-programs/

Collier, A. D. (2018). Characteristics of an effective nursing clinical instructor: The state of the science. *Journal of Clinical Nursing, 27*(1–2), 363–374. https://doi.org/10.1111/jocn.13931

Egan, K. (1978). What is curriculum? *Journal for the Canadian Association for Curriculum Studies, 9*(1), 9–16. https://jcacs.journals.yorku.ca/index.php/jcacs/article/download/16845/15651/0

Hababeh, M., & Lalithabai, D. (2020). Nurse trainees' perception of effective clinical instructor characteristics. *International Journal of Nursing Sciences, 7*(3), 285–290. https://doi.org/10.1016/j.ijstudents.2020.06.006

Jack, K., Hamshire, C., & Chambers, A. (2017). The influence of role models in undergraduate nurse education. *Journal of Clinical Nursing, 26*(23–24), 4707–4715. https://doi.org/10.1111/jocn.13822

Janse van Rensburg, E. S. (2019). Educators: Are you adequately supporting nursing students during mental health placements? *International Journal of Africa Nursing Sciences, 10,* 43–48. https://doi.org/10.1016/j.ijans.2019.01.002

Keating, S. (2015). *Curriculum development and evaluation in nursing* (3rd ed.). Springer.

Melrose, S., & Bergeron, K. (2007). Instructor immediacy strategies to facilitate group work in online graduate study. *Australasian Journal of Educational Technology, 23*(1), 132–148.

Melrose, S., Park, C., & Perry, B. (2013). *Teaching health professionals online: Frameworks and Strategies.* AU Press. https://www.aupress.ca/books/120234-teaching-health-professionals-online/

Melrose, S., Park, C., & Perry, B. (2020). *Centring human connections in the education of health professionals.* AU Press. https://www.aupress.ca/books/120289-centring-human-connections-in-the-education-of-health-professionals/

Melrose, S., Park, C., & Perry, B. (2021). *Creative clinical teaching in the health professions.* AU Press. https://www.aupress.ca/books/creative-clinical-teaching-in-the-health-professions/

Needham, J., McMurray, A., & Shaban, R. (2016). Best practice in clinical facilitation of undergraduate nursing students, *Nurse Education in Practice, 20,* 131–138. https://doi.org/10.1016/j.nepr.2016.08.003

Niederriter, E. J., Eyth, D., & Thoman, J. (2017). Nursing students' perceptions on characteristics of an effective clinical instructor. *Nursing Faculty Publications, 70.* https://engagedscholarship.csuohio.edu/nurs_facpub/70

Perry, B. (2009). Role modelling excellence in clinical nursing practice. *Nurse Education in Practice, 9*(1), 36–44. https://doi.org/10.1016/j.nepr.2008.05.001

Pringle, D., Green, L., & Johnson, S. (2004). *Nursing education in Canada: Historical review and current capacity.* Nursing Sector Study Commission. https://www.nurseone.ca/~/media/nurseone/page-content/pdf-en/nursing_education_canada_e.pdf?la=en

Reising, L. D., James, B., & Morse, B. (2018). Student perceptions of clinical instructor characteristics affecting clinical experiences. *National League of Nursing, 39*(1), 4–9. https://doi.org/10.1097/01.NEP.0000000000000241

Sadeghi, A., Oshvandi, K., & Moradi, Y. (2019). Explaining the inhibitory characteristics of clinical instructors on the process of developing clinical competence of nursing students: A qualitative study. *Journal of Family Medicine and Primary Care, 8*(5), 1664–1670. https://doi.org/10.4103/jfmpc.jfmpc_34_19

Sweet, L., & Broadbent, J. (2017). Nursing students' perceptions of the qualities of a clinical facilitator that enhance learning. *Nurse Education in Practice, 22*, 30–36. https://doi.org/10.1016/j.nepr.2016.11.007

Tuckman, B. (1965). Developmental sequence in small groups. *Psychological Bulletin, 63*(6), 384–399.

Tuckman, B., & Jensen, M. (1977). Stages of small group development. *Group and Organizational Studies, 2*(4), 419–427.

Wytenbroek, L., & Vandenberg, H. (2017). Reconsidering nursing's history during Canada 150. *Canadian Nurse, 133*(4), 120–124. https://www.canadian-nurse.com/en/articles/issues/2017/july-august-2017/reconsidering-nursings-history-during-canada-150

CHAPTER 3

Pedagogy of Clinical Teaching

Beth Perry

This chapter examines the pedagogy of clinical teaching in Canada. Strategies for establishing effective relationships with students are described; teaching and learning styles, adult education principles, lesson plan development, and learning strategies are discussed; strategies for identifying personal biases are considered; and approaches that lead to effective communication with various stakeholders are reviewed.

Chapter Outcomes

After completing the chapter, the reader will be able to
- describe strategies for establishing respectful and supportive relationships with students
- describe various teaching and learning styles, adult education principles, the development of a lesson plan, and self-directed learning approaches
- identify personal biases that may lead to premature judgement regarding student clinical performance
- identify effective communication strategies for interacting with agency and partner organization staff, patients/clients, and families to create a supportive environment for student learning

Introduction

Pedagogy is the art and science of teaching. Clinical instruction is pedagogy and clinical instructors (CIs) can hone their pedagogical abilities to create the most positive learning experiences for student nurses. While many CIs are expert nurse clinicians, there is merit in these practitioners learning specific strategies and approaches that will also make them excellent educators. In other words, some knowledge and a skill set are unique to being an exemplary pedagogue.

In this chapter, the background and history of pedagogy in clinical teaching is reviewed and specific strategies are examined that can help CIs develop respectful and supportive relationships with students. These relationships are foundational to teaching and learning success. Various teaching and learning styles are considered in conjunction with the basic principles by which adults learn best. Instruction is provided related to lesson plan development. Finally, communication strategies that CIs may find helpful as they interact with placement agencies, patients/clients, and families are identified. Throughout the chapter, emphasis is placed on the practical strategies, knowledge, skills, and self-awareness that will facilitate a nurse clinician becoming a CI who students experience as supportive, organized, knowledgeable, and effective.

Background and History of Pedagogy in Clinical Teaching

Teaching has changed over the years. The primary technology used by teachers only a few dozen years ago were chalkboards and hardcover textbooks. Today, teachers and students use mobile devices, e-books, virtual reality, and cloud storage. Increased widespread availability of technology has altered how teachers teach and how students learn. This change has also impacted the work of CIs.

The learning environment has changed from rows of desks with a teacher at the front of the class to students grouped in various ways and the teacher often acting as a "guide on the side," rather than at the front of a classroom as a "sage on the stage." Teaching is no longer considered the act of downloading knowledge into a student. Today, teaching often involves collaboration and partnerships between students and teachers. Educators pose questions, provide engaging and interactive learning activities, and guide, challenge, and support students as they become lifelong learners.

Years ago, the information on a given topic was limited. Teachers had a certain amount of content to teach. They could then assess whether they had been successful in conveying that information if students acquired that knowledge. Today, the knowledge on a given topic is nearly infinite. Teaching today focuses (at least in part) on helping students develop digital literacy and digital fluency so that they will make informed choices about which knowledge is valid and reliable. Teachers today place less emphasis on rote memorization and more on students being skilled at locating, assessing, and curating knowledge.

The compositions of the student body and teacher workforce have become more diverse. Currently, a class of students may include individuals from a variety of age groups, cultures, religions, and genders. Similarly, there is often wide diversity in teachers. Students and teachers reflect societal changes related to globalization and inclusion, a reality that makes teaching and learning today more challenging but also richer and more interesting.

Strategies for Establishing Respectful and Supportive Relationships with Students

The student-teacher relationship is an essential foundation for effective nursing education. A focus on the centrality of this relationship is continuing to emerge as we embrace new paradigms of nursing education. Successful student-teacher relationships that are experienced as supportive and respectful by both parties foster learning and transformation, especially in clinical practice settings. When students feel supported and respected by their CI, it sets the stage for a connection with the instructor that gives learners the confidence to engage fully in practice learning. Further, this connection, founded on trust and mutual respect, motivates students, helps with skill learning, decreases student stress, minimizes failure, and helps to socialize learners into their professional roles as registered nurses. A successful relationship begins when students feel supported by CIs.

Strategies Students Recognize as Supportive

When nursing students perceive the actions of CIs as supportive it has a positive impact on their relationship and on the outcomes of their learning in the clinical setting (Heydari et al., 2013). Heydari et al. (2013) identified three types of support: educational, emotional, and social. Effective educators can employ specific strategies for providing these types of support. When learners experience support, they have more self-confidence, less anxiety, and a sense of belonging in an unfamiliar clinical setting.

Educational Support

Educational support is provided by CIs to help students accomplish clinical skills by creating opportunities for them to practise these skills. Educational support includes being attuned to each student's learning goals and taking deliberate steps to match these with learning opportunities that arise, maximizing the use of educational situations. Further, when students are accompanied by a CI they perceive as supportive while they participate in these practice situations, it allows them to develop the self-confidence required to achieve learning goals. One strategy that facilitates educational support is reviewing a skill with the student before the student undertakes this skill with a patient/client. This rehearsal helps with student success in the real setting. After the student has completed the skill, a private debriefing with the individual can also facilitate learning. Another important strategy is to stay with the student during the entire skill practice opportunity. The fear of being left alone hinders the development of a sense of educational support and can negatively affect the teacher-student relationship. Simply telling a nervous student you will be present during the entire procedure can give the student added confidence.

Emotional Support

Students experience emotional support when instructors use strategies to help calm them during stressful situations. Emotional support helps to build learning confidence and guides learners to adjust and correct in a professional and appropriate way. When students feel reassured and less stressed, performance is usually enhanced.

Strategies for conveying emotional support can include talking through a skill before the student performs it and telling the student you will support them during the skill with hints and direction, if needed. Another approach is to create an atmosphere in which students feel safe verbalizing mistakes (or steps they took that were less than ideal). Encouraging students to be upfront about any errors they make also helps to protect patient/client safety. CIs who help students problem solve when an issue arises help to reduce student anxiety while protecting patient/client well-being. Students experience such instructors as emotionally supportive.

Social Support

Often, students and CIs are guests in the learning environment. Effective CIs support learners socially by easing their entry into the clinical setting. For example, a CI can introduce students to staff and facilitate positive interactions and acceptance of the students. Students often feel like strangers in a new land when they first enter a new clinical setting. Having an instructor with them provides them with an affiliate and a sense of social support until they can establish their own relationships with staff and cultivate a sense of belonging.

Social support also involves helping to develop relationships between students and patients/clients. Effective instructors help students by role modelling positive introductions and interactions with those in their care. Further, if interpersonal relationship issues or problems arise, students value instructors who stand by them and support them as they work through these challenges.

Strategies Students Recognize as Respect

Students value being respected by their instructors and link respect to feeling listened to and cared about by educators (Thompson, 2018). When respect is manifest in the student-instructor relationship, there are more positive student behaviours and improved academic performance (Thompson, 2018). Further, organizational culture and organizational processes play an important role in demonstrating to students that they are respected (Thompson, 2018). Feeling disrespected by CIs can have serious and life-changing effects on students (Hogan et al., 2019).

Respect is often conveyed in little things educators do that are really not small at all. For example, something as simple as saying hello or good morning to students and warmly greeting and acknowledging them demonstrates respect. As mentioned in Chapter 2, when CIs provide learners with timely, helpful, and sincere feedback on performance, it demonstrates that students' learning and success are important. Helping students realize what they already know and then helping them build on those existing knowledge and skills demonstrates to students that they are coming to the learning environment with a solid foundation on which to advance their competencies. When CIs acknowledge students as bringing useful prior knowledge to the clinical learning environment, it demonstrates respect for students and helps to build their confidence and increase the likelihood of success (Sybing, 2019). Helping students relate lessons learned to their own backgrounds helps students integrate learning. CIs need to know each student individually to be able to help them make connections between their own backgrounds and current learning.

Purkey's (2016) invitational education theory and practice places respect as one of the cornerstones of a successful learning environment. According to this theory, educators demonstrate respect, in part, by learning about students (including their families and hobbies), and, in turn, educators who practise invitational education disclose appropriate information about themselves (Purkey, 2016). This reciprocal exchange helps to convey respect for the individuality and humanity of each student (and teacher). Estepp and Roberts (2015) also encourage educators to relate personal experiences to the concepts being taught. When a skilled and experienced educator tells students about a relevant experience of their own at an opportune moment, it can have a profound impact on what students remember. It also conveys to students that their CI trusts and respects them. Again, what seems like a modest gesture of respect that takes little time or energy then results in large payoffs in terms of building student confidence and feelings of belonging, creating a sense of a learning community, and enhancing motivation. Teachers who are authentically inviting acknowledge that some students accept the invitation to engage in mutual sharing of personal information, and others decline it (Roe, 2019).

The Value of Connection in the Teacher-Student Relationship

When educators develop respectful and supportive relationships with students, a connection can evolve. This connection can have a positive impact on the students' clinical learning experiences and on their socialization as nurses (Gillespie, 2009). A teacher-student connection arises when the teacher conveys caring, knowing, trust, and respect and when students reciprocate by conveying similar qualities (Gillespie, 2009). In such connected relationships, students feel secure and able to focus on learning. Sybing (2019) notes that positive rapport between students and teachers results in increased learner engagement and motivation, which ultimately translate to students achieving learning outcomes.

How does a CI go about achieving a connection with students, beyond using the strategies that convey respect and support for students discussed above? Classic theorists Chickering and Gamson (1987) provide specific guidance related to pedagogies that can help achieve this connection. These pedagogies include encouraging contacts between students and teachers, using active learning strategies, communicating high expectations, and respecting diverse talents and ways of learning (Chickering & Gamson, 1987). Estepp and Roberts (2015) agree that helpful and appropriate student-teacher connections are best established when there is active involvement of students and collaboration between parties with the goal of achieving learning success.

The possibility of a useful and appropriate teacher-student connection must consider the inherent perceived power differential in the relationship. In the learning environment, students are often considered novices and teachers experts, meaning that a power differential exists. Further, teachers have the power to pass or fail a student, which potentially sets up an obstacle to building rapport. Given this reality, it becomes essential for teachers to take proactive steps to creating connections with students, and CIs can use strategies to minimize the impact of the power differential and build rapport with students. The predominant strategy educators can use to achieve this outcome is choosing communication approaches that convey genuine interest and willing investment in student success. The profession of nursing focuses on interpersonal relationships. To help nursing students become skilled at human interaction, nurse educators need to consciously model effective communication skills as part of their pedagogy, both to teach communication skills and to create connections with students that facilitate clinical teaching success.

Teaching and Learning Styles

How can we teach students if we do not know how they learn? Recognizing that teaching and learning styles help determine suitable instructional approaches is important for CIs to succeed. It is commonly accepted that students have individual preferences in terms of how they learn best. Often, students have a dominant learning style, and if CIs can match their teaching strategies to that learner's preferred style, the likelihood that the student will achieve competencies increases. Further, an appropriate matching of learning and teaching styles can have positive outcomes for educators and for students. Education based on learning styles enhances students' academic achievement and teachers' professional satisfaction (Vizeshfar & Torabizadeh, 2018).

Simply, an individual's learning style refers to the way in which the student prefers to or is best able to absorb, process, comprehend, and retain information. The most common model of learning styles is the VARK model of student learning (Fleming & Mills, 1992). The acronym VARK stands for four learning styles: visual, auditory, reading/writing, and kinesthetic (Fleming & Mills, 1992). Sometimes, the reading/writing preference is omitted and then it is referred to as the VAK model. Visual learners learn best when pictures, graphics, mind maps, and other images are used in instruction. Auditory learners learn by listening and speaking and enjoy lectures and small group discussions. Students who fall into the reading and writing preference style are often note takers and enjoy readings as they learn from words. Finally, kinesthetic learners are hands-on learners and learn best by physically doing a task or manipulating objects that represent concepts.

While the VARK Model remains the standard for differentiating learning styles, there are likely many additional learning style schemes (Pashler et al., 2009). Despite all the possible variations in learning styles, the basic principle is that each person has a way or ways they learn best. The message for CIs is that "optimal instruction requires diagnosing individuals' learning style[s] and tailoring instruction accordingly" (Pashler et al., 2009, p. 105).

While knowing which learning style a student prefers is helpful to CIs because they can align the curriculum (and individual learning strategies) to match the preferred style, some students have multiple preferred learning modes. Additionally, if a class has students from all four preferred modes of learning, CIs may need to offer a choice of learning options so that students can access alternatives that suit their style(s). Being aware of various learning styles and making options available will increase students' levels of comprehension, motivation, confidence, and metacognition (Fleming & Mills, 1992).

CIs should be aware that their own preferred learning style may influence how they approach teaching (D'Angelo et al., 2019). In other words, as teachers, visual learners may lean towards instructional approaches that primarily focus on using infographics and mind maps to guide student learning. A kinesthetic learner may adopt a teaching philosophy that encourages students to learn to do by doing. Self-awareness becomes important, as does knowing your tendencies and appreciating that not all students share your learning (and teaching) style preference. Some theorists promote the idea that educators should develop a repertoire of styles so that they can adapt their teaching approaches to accommodate the learning style preference of the student they are instructing.

Adult Education Principles

Adult learners often share some commonalities, and recognizing this can facilitate student success. For example, adults often bring important life experiences with them to their learning situations. These experiences will vary from person to person and create a diverse population in a single class. A certain level of maturity and confidence commonly arise from having lived life outside the classroom. Adult learning theory posits that adult students can direct their learning experience and use life experiences to aid in the learning process (Knowles, 1975). This often results in adult students who are self-directed and who bring a sense of partnership to the teacher-student relationship (Ross-Gordon, 2011). In other words, adult students come with certain skills, knowledge, and attitudes that can often be a solid foundation for further learning. Additionally, they may respond best to CIs who respect their existing competencies and partner with them on the learning journey. Providing mature students with the opportunity to be self-directed and to make choices that help them achieve their specific learning needs (using their preferred learning styles) is a powerful strategy for CIs to consider.

Adult learning is sometimes called *andragogy* (as opposed to *pedagogy* or the teaching of children). Knowles et al. (2005) specified five principles of andragogy:
- Adult learners take responsibility for their own learning.
- Life experiences are an important foundation to further learning.
- Learning for adults needs to be practical and applicable.
- Learners need to know why they need to learn something.
- Adult learners are internally motivated to achieve learning goals.

Additionally, some adults may fear failure in part because they have faced criticism and rejection in the past. Teachers need to be aware that adult students may be anxious and need encouragement and recognition of their achievements. In short, adult learners need teachers who believe they can succeed. One strategy CIs can use is to help students set short-term achievable learning goals early in the learning experience. Achieving these can increase student confidence and set the student up for success. Authentic, supportive, and swift feedback from instructors is highly valued by adult students.

Further, adult students appreciate a learning challenge. This helps to sustain their interest and build their confidence as they are asked to push their learning and skills to new levels. CIs must find the balance between challenging students too far beyond their abilities (in which case students may give up and sense failure) and under challenging them, which can feel insulting and results in students who are bored and unmotivated. One of the most satisfying moments for CIs and student alike is succeeding in a challenge.

Adult students have likely engaged in several learning situations before coming to the current learning environment. Because of this history, adults bring with them expectations about teaching and learning. These students may have spoken and unspoken expectations of their CIs, and a frank and open conversation with students at the outset can be helpful to both parties. One expectation adult students usually have is that what they learn will be immediately useful. They often have little time or respect for learning that will not have practical application to their real-world work or life. For example, they will be more engaged in learning a skill that they can use to improve patient care or to acquire a new work role or promotion. Adults appreciate content that is directly relevant to their own learning goals. CIs can invite students to engage in self-assessment of their existing competencies and then tailor learning experiences to help students achieve their self-identified learning gaps. Treating adult learners as responsible people who have a vested and genuine interest in their learning and personal growth usually nets positive outcomes. Involving adults in all aspects of their learning from determining learning goals to choosing learning activities to achieve those goals demonstrates the respect that adult learners appreciate.

The Development of a Lesson Plan

A road map is essential for reaching a destination. In teaching, this road map is commonly called a lesson plan. Lesson plans usually include learning goals and strategies for achieving those goals. Skilled adult educators collaborate with students in developing lesson plans targeted to the learning goals, preferred learning styles, and types of learning activities most effective for specific learners.

A successful lesson plan addresses and integrates three key components:
- learning outcomes
- learning activities
- strategies for evaluation of achievement of learning outcomes

Learning Outcomes

Learning outcomes are what the student will achieve (know or be able to do) because of successfully completing the learning activities. Alternatively, a learning objective is what the teacher will do to help the student achieve the learning outcomes. In other words, an outcome is student focused and an objective is instructor focused. Effective learning outcomes begin with a carefully selected verb of the appropriate level (i.e., describe, analyze, evaluate). Effective learning outcomes are achievable, can be demonstrated or measured, and describe important learning goals.

Benjamin Bloom (1956) published *Taxonomy of Educational Objectives*, commonly known as Bloom's taxonomy (see Figure 3.1). Bloom's taxonomy is the framework used by generations of educators as they created learning outcomes in three domains: cognitive, psychomotor, and affective. Each category contains subcategories lying along a continuum from simple to complex and concrete to abstract. More recently, Bloom's revised taxonomy of educational objectives (Anderson & Krathwohl, 2001) was developed and is useful to educators who are setting learning outcomes.

Figure 3.1 Bloom's Taxonomy

Bloom's Taxonomy

- **create** — Produce new or original work
  Design, assemble, construct, conjecture, develop, formulate, author, investigate
- **evaluate** — Justify a stand or decision
  appraise, argue, defend, judge, select, support, value, critique, weigh
- **analyze** — Draw connections among ideas
  differentiate, organize, relate, compare, contrast, distinguish, examine, experiment, question, test
- **apply** — Use information in new situations
  execute, implement, solve, use, demonstrate, interpret, operate, schedule, sketch
- **understand** — Explain ideas or concepts
  classify, describe, discuss, explain, identify, locate, recognize, report, select, translate
- **remember** — Recall facts and basic concepts
  define, duplicate, list, memorize, repeat, state

Vanderbilt University Center for Teaching

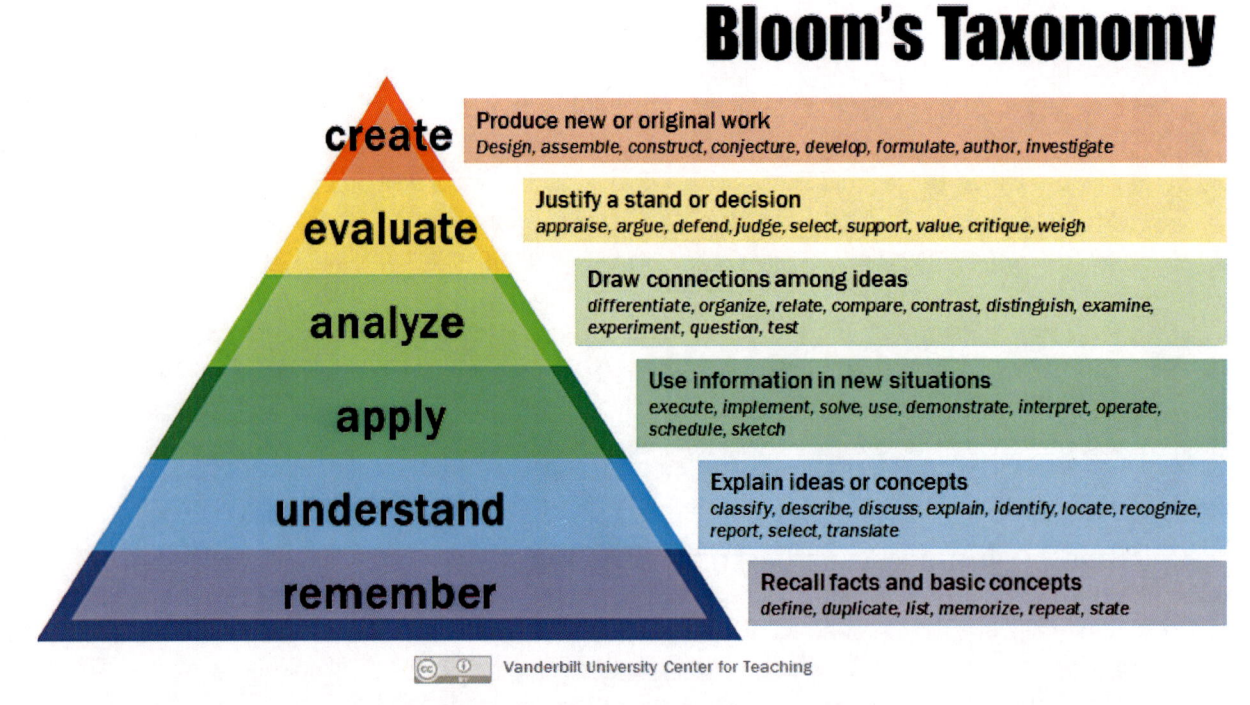

Source: From Vanderbilt University Center for Teaching (2021).

Learning to craft learning outcomes that are at the appropriate level and meet the other criteria for well-developed learning outcomes is a skill CIs need to develop. It takes considerable practice to become effective at developing learning outcomes. Many online resources are available (i.e., Bloom's taxonomy verb tables, worksheets to guide learning outcome writing), and educators are encouraged to consult these if they are required to develop learning outcomes for students they are instructing.

Learning Activities

An educator's priority is to make sure learning activities address learning outcomes. When learning activities are not geared to achieving learning outcomes, learners become frustrated, and needed learning goals are not achieved. It can be effective to begin with the end in mind. Collaborate with adult students and be clear on what students need to be able to do, think, know, and value by the end of the learning experience. These are the learning outcomes. Next, consider how these ends can be achieved. These are the learning activities. Keep in mind the learning style preferences of each student and match them to learning opportunities (activities) to help each student achieve the desired outcomes. It is essential to match learning activities to the learning domains (cognitive, psychomotor, affective) and to the level within the domain. For example, if a learning outcome is a cognitive domain learning outcome, and the level of thinking is applied, then an appropriate learning activity might include demonstrating a procedure or having students practise using a new intravenous pump. If the cognitive domain learning outcome level of thinking is in the remember category, then appropriate learning activities include listing the side effects of a specific medication or repeating the steps for starting an intravenous (see Figure 3.1).

If learning activities are matched to the learning outcome and matched again to the domain (and level with the domain) then learners should achieve the stated learning outcomes. It is important that the learning outcomes can be measured (or otherwise evaluated) to ensure that they have been achieved.

Self-Directed Learning Approaches

Self-directedness is considered appropriate for adult students as they take responsibility for their own learning, both in the present and for future professional development. Knowles (1975) defined self-directed learning as a process in which individuals determine their own learning needs, formulate learning goals, decide on resources and strategies to meet their learning needs, and evaluate the learning outcomes. Self-directed learning enables nursing students to evolve into lifelong learners who are skilled at knowing what they do not know and knowing how to learn what they need to through strategies that are appropriate to their learning style.

CIs need to cultivate a skill set in student nurses that includes self-motivation, self-management, self-monitoring, self-control, and reflection. These skills are fostered when educators show genuine interest and care towards students and regard for their learning (Jasmi & Hin, 2014). In other words, a positive teacher-student relationship sets a foundation for the nurturing of self-directedness in students.

Living in a digital age may enhance the possibility of self-direction in learning. Having constant access to the internet has changed how students seek new knowledge, store information, and share opinions and reflections. Students no longer depend on an assigned teacher as their only source of knowledge and evaluator of learning. Rather, students have access to skilled teachers (and some not so skilled) from around the world at a click of a button. Further, knowledge is delivered to their phones and computers instantly and in the form that matches their preferred learning styles (video, audio, graphics etc.). Because students are living in a digital reality, teachers need to teach digital literacy and fluency as these are foundation to students being capable, self-directed learners.

Personal Biases and Premature Judgement of Student Clinical Performance

The education of health professionals depends on interpersonal interactions that are particularly susceptible to the positive and negative effects of teacher bias. Personal biases can make you less effective as an educator. In particular, your ability to communicate with and evaluate students can be impeded by biases—some that you may not even be aware of. For example, biases can result in premature judgements that can have a negative effect on accurate student assessment. Your biases may be based on very superficial student qualities such as physical appearance, way of speaking, family situation, gender, quirks, attire, mannerisms, or age—all factors that should not influence your disposition towards a student.

A bias may predispose you to treat students unfairly. A positive bias may mean you don't see a student's weaknesses while a negative bias may result in you negatively evaluating a student's academic performance without cause. Recognizing your personal predisposition to certain biases is the first step in preventing the unwanted and unjust effects on students and their achievements.

How can CIs become more aware of their subconscious associations and prevent premature judgement of student performance in a clinical setting? First, recognize that your assumptions about students with certain qualities are probably a result of prior experiences or interactions that you are now applying to this student. Deliberately reflect on your views about certain students, determining which qualities you find appealing and which you find off-putting. Ask yourself the following questions:

- Which students do you naturally respond to in a more positive or negative way?
- Which students do you tend to spend more time with?
- Which students do you look forward to having conversation with or to helping with a clinical skill?
- Do you see any trends in terms of which traits you find appealing and which qualities you find unsettling, challenging, or objectionable?
- Do you find yourself most comfortable with students who are like you in certain ways?

This honest self-reflection is an important starting point. If you find yourself reacting in an especially positive or negative way to a student, challenge yourself to consider whether your reaction is warranted or whether a bias is colouring your approach.

If you can be honest with yourself about your biases, you can take action to avoid the systematic judgement error that can result. Becoming aware of your ingrained biases can help prevent you from making unfair presumptions that can impact interpersonal relationships, impair learning, reduce the fairness of assessment, and create a toxic learning environment. In particular, if students sense that you are treating them or others unfairly, it can have a negative impact on their level of trust. Trust is a foundational pillar to creating an effective and inviting learning environment (Purkey, 2016). Perceived unfairness can lead to students becoming disengaged in learning and can add a psychological burden that negatively impacts learning (Elks et al., 2020).

A more universal strategy that educators can use to minimize the potential effects of bias is to practice empathy towards all learners. Adopting a teaching philosophy some call a *pedagogy of kindness* means (in part) that you make efforts to understand all students' emotions and perspectives. A pedagogy of kindness is a teaching philosophy that is guided by kindness, compassion, and care (Serbati et al., 2020). The use of kindness, which includes care and empathy as a teaching strategy, can positively influence learning environments and student outcomes. CIs who have the capacity to identify with students and who form strong teacher-student relationships have a positive impact on learners' feelings of self-worth, and these instructors can favourably influence learners' academic achievements (Serbati et al., 2020). An initial step in becoming empathetic is using deliberate strategies to get to know students, including a little about their personal life circumstances and their interests, values, and priorities.

All educators are human and prone to behaving in a certain way towards others based (at least in part) on characteristics or qualities that may be beyond their control. Biases are normal, but if you do not take steps to become self-aware and guard against their intrusion on your teaching and on the learning environment, biases can be very destructive and hamper student achievement. If you do take bias recognition and control seriously, it can improve your connections with students and help you make clear and honest assessments of their learning.

Communication Strategies Essential for Clinical Educators

As mentioned, excellent interpersonal communication skills are essential for CI success. Educators spend much of their time on communication activities. CIs need to interact with learners, agency and institutional staff, and patients/clients and their family members. Being an effective CI can be intellectually and emotional demanding, in part because of the nature of the work and the work environment. You are responsible not only for the education of a new generation of nurses but also for the lives of vulnerable people. Your ability to communicate effectively in emotion-filled, chaotic, noisy, and sometimes urgent situations is a major challenge of your role. An entire book could be devoted to essential communication strategies for CIs. In this section, the essential strategies are summarized.

Clarity

Make sure you communicate what you really mean to say. It may seem elementary, but unclear or ambiguous messages can be misinterpreted, and conflict or harmful misunderstandings result that can damage relationships. To be clear, take time to carefully construct important messages and review them (at least in your mind) to see where misinterpretation may occur. Reframe your messages until you are sure they say exactly what you intend. Poor word choice, uncontrolled vocal inflection, or incongruent body language can hamper the clarity of your comments. Most importantly, check with the person you are communicating with to ensure they heard not only your words but also the intention behind your message.

Compassion

There will be times when what is most important in your communication is that you convey compassion. The student who has just experienced their first patient death, the learner who has been confronted by an angry physician, the family member who is confused about visitor regulations, the agency manager who does not want any students on the unit—these are all situations in which your communication skills will be tested. If you are unsure begin by being compassionate. Try to put yourself for a moment in the position of the other person. How are they feeling? What can you say to avoid putting them on the defensive? Often, a comment or question in which the person can sense your compassion and caring can help to diffuse the situation and open the possibility of helpful dialogue.

Empowerment

As a CI, you are in a position of power, especially with students. Your words matter. Carefully chosen and timely words of encouragement, praise, or acknowledgement can have a profound impact on student competence, self-determination, and confidence. Empowering messages can inspire students to take initiative, reduce their stress, and help them to believe in themselves (Berkovich & Eyal, 2018). CIs also empower others when they demonstrate involvement in the conversation through appropriate eye contact, gestures, paraphrasing, and questioning (Bjekić et al., 2020). If you show engagement in a conversation, it conveys that the other is important to you and that you value what they have to say.

Emotional Expressivity and Sensitivity

Bjekić et al. (2020) conclude that effective communicators can display emotions, attitudes, and feelings appropriately during human interactions. Likewise, skilled communicators are sensitive to the verbal and non-verbal messages of others by noticing, receiving, and interpreting what others are trying to communicate (Bjekić et al., 2020). This communication skill may seem suspect to some educators. It may seem more important to maintain control, detachment, and neutrality in interactions with the various stakeholders who educators must communicate with. While maintaining a positive and professional tone is essential; truly effective educators are not afraid to share their humanity in certain situations. For example, letting a traumatized student know that you also made a medication error in your past and that you were terrified to admit it to your teacher can teach a student valuable lessons in owning up to errors and learning from mistakes. Crying with a family member who just lost a loved one whom one of your students was caring for role models compassion for the student.

A CI's skill in human-to-human communication has an impact on the teaching process, students' achievements, and relationships with essential stakeholders. Development of communication competence requires ongoing professional development on the part of the teacher.

Summary

CIs can hone their pedagogical knowledge and skills to create positive learning experiences for student nurses. Clinical education has become increasingly dependent on technology, and today CIs engage with students to identify learning needs and discover ways to meet the learning goals of increasingly diverse students. Skilled CIs use deliberate strategies for building relationships with students that students perceive as supportive and respectful. Successful CIs consider their own teaching style and the learning style of students and apply principles of adult education as they craft lesson plans and develop learning activities students find challenging and engaging. Self-reflection related to personal biases that may result in premature judgement of a student's actions and interactions is a critical skill for CIs. Finally, learning effective communication strategies is foundational to CI success.

Conclusion

This chapter examined the pedagogy of clinical teaching in Canada. Strategies for establishing effective relationships with students were described; teaching and learning styles, adult education principles, lesson plan development, and learning strategies were discussed; strategies for identifying personal biases were considered; and approaches that can lead to effective communication with various stakeholders were reviewed. Becoming an excellent CI takes experience, honest self-reflection, commitment to continual improvement, and a desire to motivate and nurture beginning nurses. Being a CI is hard work, but doing it well can be intensely rewarding—for you and for the students you inspire.

References

Anderson, L. W., & Krathwohl, D. R. (2001). *A taxonomy for learning, teaching, and assessing* (abridged ed.). Allyn & Bacon.

Berkovich, I., & Eyal, O. (2018). Principals' emotional support and teachers' emotional reframing: The mediating role of principals' supportive communication strategies. *Psychology in the Schools, 55*(7), 867–879. https://doi.org/10.1002/pits.22130

Bjekić, D., Zlatić, L., & Bojović, M. (2020). Students-teachers' communication competence: Basic social communication skills and interaction involvement. *Journal of Educational Sciences & Psychology, 10*(1), 24–34.

Bloom, B. S., Engelhart, M. D., Furst, E. J., Hill, W. H., & Krathwohl, D. R. (Eds.). (1956). *Taxonomy of educational objectives: The classification of educational goals; Handbook I: Cognitive domain*. David McKay.

Chickering, A. W., & Gamson, Z. F. (1987). Seven principles for good practice in undergraduate education. *American Association for Higher Education, 39*(7), 3–7.

D'Angelo, T., Harsh, J., Bunch, J. C., Lamm, A., Thoron, A., & Roberts, G. (2019). Exploring learning styles expressed in teaching philosophies among agriculture university teaching faculty. *Journal of Agricultural Education, 1*, 283. https://doi.org/10.5032/jae.2019.01283

Elks, M. L., Johnson, K., & Anachebe, N. F. (2020). Morehouse School of Medicine case study: Teacher-learner relationships free of bias and discrimination. *Academic Medicine, 95*(12S), S88–S92. https://doi.org/10.1097/ACM.0000000000003678

Estepp, C. M., & Roberts, T. G. (2015). Teacher immediacy and professor/student rapport as predictors of motivation and engagement. *NACTA Journal, 59*(2), 155–163.

Fleming, N., & Mills, C. (1992). Not another inventory, rather a catalyst for reflection. *To Improve the Academy, 11*(1), 137–148. https://doi.org/10.1002/j.2334-4822.1992.tb00213.x

Gillespie, C. M. (2009). The essence of student-teacher connection in the student-teacher relationship in clinical nursing education. *Journal of Advanced Nursing, 37*(6), 566–576. https://doi.org/10.1046/j.1365-2648.2002.02131.x

Heydari, A., Yaghoubinia, R., & Roudsari, R. (2013). Supportive relationship: Experiences of Iranian students and teachers concerning student-teacher relationship in clinical nursing education. *Iranian Journal of Nursing and Midwifery Research, 18*(6), 467–474.

Hogan, T., Ricci, C., & Ryan, T. (2019). Respecting students: Abusive classroom teacher verbal behaviour. *Journal of Pedagogical Research, 3*(3), 151–165. https://doi.org/10.33902/jpr.v3i3.139

Knowles, M. (1975). *Self-directed learning: A guide for learners and teachers*. Association Press.

Knowles, M. S., Holton, E. F., & Swanson, R. A. (2005). *The adult learner: The definitive classic in adult education and human resource development*. Elsevier.

Pashler, H., McDaniel, M., Rohrer, D., & Bjork, R. (2009). Learning styles: Concepts and evidence. *Psychological Science in the Public Interest, 9*(3), 103–119.

Purkey, W. W. (2016). *History of the International Alliance for Invitational Education*. https://www.invitationaleducation.org/iaie/history

Jasmi, A., & Hin, L. (2014). Student-teacher relationship and student academic motivation. *Journal of Interdisciplinary Research in Education, 4*(1), 75–82.

Roe, K. (2019). Supporting student assets and demonstrating respect for funds of knowledge. *Journal of Invitational Theory and Practice, 25*, 5–13.

Ross-Gordon, J. M. (2011). Research on adult learners: Supporting the needs of a student population that is no longer non-traditional. *Peer Review, 13*(1), 26–29.

Serbati, A., Aquario, D., Da Re, L., Paccagnella, O., & Felisatti, E. (2020). Exploring good teaching practices and needs for improvement: Implications for staff development. *Journal of Educational, Cultural and Psychological Studies (ECPS Journal),* (21), 43–64. https://doi.org/10.7358/ecps-2020-021-serb

Sybing, R. (2019). Making connections: Student-teacher rapport in higher education classrooms. *Journal of the Scholarship of Teaching and Learning, 19*(5), 18–35.

Thompson, C. S. (2018). The construct of "respect" in teacher-student relationships: Exploring dimensions of ethics of care and sustainable development. *Journal of Leadership Education, 17*(3), 42–60.

Vanderbilt University Center for Teaching. (2021). *Bloom's cognitive domain.* https://cft.vanderbilt.edu/guides-sub-pages/blooms-taxonomy/

Vizeshfar, F., & Torabizadeh, C. (2018). The effect of teaching based on dominant learning style on nursing students' academic achievement. *Nurse Education in Practice, 28,* 103–108. https://doi.org/10.1016/j.nepr.2017.10.013

CHAPTER 4

Fostering the Development of Clinical Judgement and Reasoning

Patrick Lavoie & Marie-France Deschênes

This chapter examines the pedagogy of clinical judgement and reasoning in the clinical setting. First, the concepts of clinical judgement and clinical reasoning are distinguished. Next, an overview of the evidence regarding these concepts is presented and they are conceptualized as components of clinical competence, which develops throughout a nurse's career. Principles of effective supervision of clinical judgement and reasoning are then discussed. Finally, practical strategies for assisting students with clinical judgement and reasoning difficulties are identified.

Chapter Objectives

After completing the chapter, the reader will be able to
- differentiate the concepts of clinical judgement and clinical reasoning
- recognize the context-bound, holistic, and developmental characteristics of clinical judgement and reasoning
- describe the principles of effective supervision of clinical judgement and reasoning
- identify practical strategies to assist students with clinical judgement and reasoning difficulties

Introduction

Thinking back on his early days working in the intensive care unit, Patrick recalls a charge nurse telling him that critical care nursing required excellent clinical judgement.

"But what is clinical judgement?" he asked.

"Clinical judgement is knowing not to give beta-blockers to a patient with chronic obstructive pulmonary disease," she answered.

As for Marie-France, when she began supervising nursing students, she remembers hearing some colleagues say, "Either students have clinical judgement, or they don't have it at all." This left her to wonder, *Are there ways to help students develop their clinical judgement and reasoning?*

Clinical judgement and reasoning are two of the most fundamental concepts in nursing education and practice. After all, they both refer to the wisdom and intelligence that characterize seasoned nurses. Although most know what these terms refer to, it is often difficult to articulate clear definitions. It can be easier to recognize poor clinical judgement or reasoning than to describe the opposite. The challenge is even greater when it comes to guiding students in developing their clinical judgement and reasoning. What should a clinical instructor (CI) pay attention to in the clinical setting? What questions should be asked? How do we help students as they progress towards expertise—and what happens when a student struggles?

This chapter presents an overview of what every CI should know to support students in developing their clinical judgement and reasoning in the clinical setting. Following a brief overview of conceptual and theoretical foundations, clinical judgement and reasoning are discussed as components of clinical competence, which develops throughout a nurse's career. Principles of effective supervision of clinical judgement and reasoning are then considered. Finally, practical strategies for assisting students with clinical judgement and reasoning difficulties are identified. Throughout the chapter, emphasis is placed on the positive impact that a CI's commitment to students' learning may have on them becoming effective practitioners.

Background and History

Many expressions are used to discuss how nurses think in the clinical setting. Concepts such as *clinical reasoning*, *clinical judgement*, *decision-making*, and *critical thinking* are often used interchangeably, as well as in other combinations, such as *critical judgement* or *clinical thinking*. Nevertheless, it is essential to differentiate these terms because they represent different but related phenomena.

Definitions

Clinical judgement is the output of a nurse's thought process. According to Tanner (2006), a clinical judgement can take the form of an assessment or a conclusion about a patient's health, concerns, or needs. It can also take the form of a decision to act (or not to act) and the choice of an intervention approach. For example, concluding that a patient is in pain and deciding to administer an analgesic are two clinical judgements that nurses make regularly.

Clinical reasoning is the thought process that precedes a clinical judgement (Tanner, 2006). Like any process, it implies that some input is transformed through a series of activities. In the case of clinical reasoning, the input is a set of data, which is transformed into a clinical judgement through various cognitive processes. For example, a student who observes that a post-operative patient is grimacing may recognize pain but will need to ask additional questions and examine the patient to collect and analyze data to understand the source and nature of this pain. An experienced nurse may recognize pain more intuitively and expedite the clinical reasoning process, collecting less data and understanding what is going on more rapidly. In both cases, a set of data (input) is transformed into a judgement (output) through a series of analytic or intuitive processes, depending on the nurse's knowledge base, experience, and expertise.

Clinical decision-making and *critical thinking* are more general and encompassing concepts that are sometimes criticized for their lack of specificity (Monteiro et al., 2020). The former represents the continual and contextual process of gathering, interpreting, and evaluating clinical data to select an evidence-based choice of action (Tiffen et al., 2014). Accordingly, it describes both the process (reasoning) and the output (judgement) of the nursing thinking process. The latter is often described as a generic set of cognitive skills (i.e., interpretation, analysis, inference, explanation, evaluation, self-regulation) and affective dispositions (i.e., open-minded, inquisitive, truth-seeking, analytical, systematic, self-confident) that characterize habits of the mind (Simpson & Courtney, 2002). Therefore, critical thinking applies to both clinical and non-clinical contexts.

Evidence Related to Clinical Judgement and Reasoning

In this chapter, the term *clinical reasoning* describes the cognitive process that leads nurses to reach *clinical judgements*, whether these judgements are impressions about a patient's health or decisions regarding actions to be carried out. As discussed by Monteiro et al. (2020), the two concepts have been the topic of much research since the 1970s, when the functioning of the human mind was first compared to an information processing system much like a computer. Researchers believed that clinical reasoning relied on cognitive strategies to process and analyze data collected by the five senses. Consequently, they became interested in identifying these strategies so that they could be taught to students.

Studies conducted at the time showed that both novice and expert clinicians used similar cognitive strategies. When facing a clinical problem, they quickly generated tentative hypotheses to explain the information at hand and collected additional data to either confirm or refute these hypotheses. Such an analytic process is often called the hypothetico-deductive method. The only difference was that experts generated better hypotheses than did novices. It was also shown that the accumulation of experience accelerated clinicians' reasoning and improved their capacity to recognize typical clinical patterns. The concept of intuition is often used to describe this capacity of expert nurses to know instantly what is going on with a patient, sometimes without being able to explain why (Melin-Johastudentson et al., 2017). Today, most researchers acknowledge that the mind employs both analytical and intuitive reasoning. Dual-process theories of reasoning suggest that most judgements are the result of both modes of reasoning operating concurrently, depending on the demands of a situation (Evans & Stanovich, 2013).

Another stream of research focused on the role of knowledge in decision-making, rather than the strategies or skills involved in information processing (Monteiro et al., 2020). Researchers were interested in the form and structure of knowledge that is stored in the mind. They showed that compared to novices, experienced clinicians mastered a greater repertoire of knowledge, which was more organized and connected. Concepts such as *prototypes*, *exemplars*, and *scripts* have emerged from this work. Based on this research, a nurse's mind can be compared not only to a computer that processes information but also to a library where knowledge is stored and organized for retrieval when needed. The knowledge in a nurse's "library" can take different forms. According to Tanner (2006), theoretical or textbook knowledge is more abstract, is based on science, and can be generalized and applied in a variety of situations. Practical or experiential knowledge is knowledge that accumulates through experience in the field. Knowledge of the patient is a particular type of experiential knowledge that nurses construct through sustained engagement and interaction with patients. This type of knowledge may focus on the typical responses of a certain population of patients (e.g., patients with a chronic obstructive pulmonary disorder, mothers after childbirth) or the patterns of response, preferences, and values of an individual. In both cases, knowledge of the patient helps to individualize care.

In the clinical setting, clinical judgement and reasoning are closely tied to health assessment. Health assessment is the process by which nurses collect objective data through inspection, palpation, auscultation, or percussion, and collects subjective data through questioning and interviewing a patient (Jarvis, 2018). Such data are the raw materials from which clinical reasoning can operate. It comes from many sources, such as the patient, their relatives, the medical record, fellow nurses, and other health care professionals. As soon as nurses start to collect data, they reason and make clinical judgements. What are the priorities? What data must be collected? Which data are important and must be attended to—sometimes called *relevant cues*? Which data are less important and can be overlooked or dealt with later? All these judgements result from clinical reasoning, which operates at the interface of the nurse's knowledge and the patient's situation.

But that is not all. In addition to their knowledge, nurses' backgrounds influence their clinical judgement and reasoning. In the clinical judgement model, Tanner (2006) suggests that a nurse's philosophy, beliefs, and values are influential, as well as their ability to engage and establish a caring relationship with the patient. For example, two nurses may have very different beliefs and values regarding pain management, which will influence their decision threshold for administering pain medication. Furthermore, the setting in which clinical judgement and reasoning occur is influential, particularly because of its cultural, political, and social characteristics. These elements combine into a set of norms, habits, and routines that determine the types of judgements nurses are expected to make and how they are to interact with each other, with patients, and with other health care professionals. Just think of the care of Indigenous people in Canada, which depends not only on the judgements of individual nurses but also on the biases and inequities embedded in the Canadian health care system. Although beyond the scope of this chapter, it is essential to understand that clinical judgement and reasoning are influenced by multiple factors beyond the nurse, the patient, and their relationship.

When the nurse has reached one or many conclusions—that is, judgements—about a patient's health, concerns, or needs, the nurse can make decisions on the interventions to respond appropriately. Once again, these decisions will be based on and evolve according to the nurse's clinical judgement and reasoning. Throughout their response, the nurse continually assesses the patient's reaction and adjusts the plan accordingly.

Thus, clinical judgement and reasoning are integral to the work of nurses in the clinical setting, from their assessment of patient situations to their decisions about a course of action and continual adaptations based on observed reactions. By now, you probably appreciate the complexity and ubiquity of clinical judgement and reasoning in nursing. It may appear to be quite a challenge for students to develop the knowledge, skills, and attitudes required for sound clinical judgement and reasoning. It might even be overwhelming to think about the kind of support they need to build those assets in the clinical setting. The next section provides some guidance regarding these points.

Clinical Competence, Judgement, and Reasoning

From an educational standpoint, clinical judgement and reasoning can be understood as two facets of a nurse's clinical competence. Although various conceptions prevail, competence can be defined as a "context-bound, holistic combination of knowledge, skills, attitudes, and values" (Charette et al., 2020, p. 2811). This means that competence is always tied to the context in which it is exercised. For example, a nurse may have excellent clinical judgement and reasoning when working with oncology patients but will likely be challenged if asked to work in a neonatal unit. Furthermore, this means that nurses must acquire and master a wide variety of resources that they must mobilize effectively to exercise their clinical judgement and reasoning. It is one thing to know the side effects of anticoagulation (knowledge), to know the technique of injecting an anticoagulant (skill), and behave in a caring manner (attitude). It is quite another to be able to mobilize and combine these individual resources and act competently and effectively when caring for a patient at an anticoagulation clinic. This is one reason that the clinical setting presents such great opportunities for the development of students' clinical judgement and reasoning.

An additional characteristic of competence is its developmental and evolutive character. Since the seminal work of Benner (1984) on nursing expertise, many educators believe that nurses progress on a path from novice to expert throughout their career. When starting nursing school, novices have a very limited set of resources and often rely on rules and procedures to decide on their actions. Throughout their education and clinical experiences, they construct an ever-growing repertoire of knowledge, skills, and attitudes that they gradually learn to mobilize effectively, in response to various clinical situations. Eventually, they move from the novice to the advanced beginner level, obtain their nursing licence, and begin working autonomously in the clinical setting, where they can gradually progress through the levels of competence and proficiency described in Benner's model. At the expert level, nurses have an intuitive grasp and comprehensive understanding of clinical situations, are flexible in their ability to adapt to diverse circumstances, and act as resources for their colleagues. Although it is purported to develop through experience, the relationship between expertise and experience is far from linear. Some nurses will reach the expert level five years after graduation, while others will never go beyond the advanced beginner level—even after 25 years of experience. For experience to foster expertise, nurses must evolve in a context that encourages reflecting, questioning, and learning from their practice and that provides opportunities to refine, hone, and expand their knowledge, skills, and attitudes (Tanner, 2006).

Building on this conception of clinical judgement and reasoning as a context-bound, holistic, and developmental competence, researchers have continued to study how nurses progress at different stages of their careers. Recently, Boyer et al. (2015) proposed a cognitive learning model of clinical judgement and reasoning in a three-year undergraduate bachelor of nursing program. This model is relevant to clinical teaching. Based on empirical observations, this model characterizes the clinical competence of students at different stages of their education and identifies the milestones that are essential to their development (see Figure 4.1). Knowing what stage of education students are at can be helpful in clinical teaching. A CI's interventions will be more effective if consistent with students' needs and progression in the development of their competence. It is also important that the CI adapts their expectancies to the competence level of the students—it would be rather unfair to expect first-year students to consider the peculiarities of a patient's environment when they are focused on learning how to collect disease-specific data in a step-by-step manner.

Figure 4.1 Characteristics of Students' Clinical Judgement and Reasoning in a Three-Year Undergraduate Bachelor of Nursing Program

Stage of education	Characteristics of clinical judgement and reasoning
Beginning (first year)	• Procedural, proceeds in a step-by-step manner: data are collected first, then analyzed, and finally acted upon • Focused on collecting objective data regarding the patient's disease • Based on theoretical and textbook knowledge, with little consideration of the peculiarities of the situation
Halfway (second year)	• More comprehensive, aimed at prioritizing and finding relevant data • Focused on data analysis, with iterations and interactions with data collection • Increased attention to other dimensions of the patient's situation (e.g., psychosocial, ethical) and subjective data • Awareness of the peculiarities of a patient's situation
End (third year)	• Dynamic; data collection, analysis, and intervention are constantly feeding into and influencing each other • More comprehensive view of the situation, prioritization of needs, and integration—rather than isolation—of various dimensions • Contextualized, considers the perspective of the patient and characteristics of their environment • Relies on various sources to enhance analysis

Source: Adapted from a figure in Boyer et al. (2015).

Clinical Teaching for Clinical Judgement and Reasoning

The clinical setting is one of the most fertile environments to foster the development of clinical judgement and reasoning. This is where students encounter authentic clinical situations and are exposed to the complexity of nursing practice. For students, every clinical situation is a learning opportunity. For CIs, observing and questioning students as they interact with a patient allows CIs to validate how students are adapting to the situation.

Yet clinical teaching for clinical judgement and reasoning is not without its challenges (Audétat et al., 2017a; Audétat et al., 2013). CIs must continually assess and adapt to the learning needs and challenges of students while keeping in mind the quality of care and patient safety. This requires not only clinical vigilance but also pedagogical competence to implement the principles of clinical judgement and reasoning supervision, detect students' difficulties, and implement remedial measures, if necessary.

Cognitive Companionship

As explained above, the development of clinical judgement and reasoning occurs over time through various opportunities for learning by experience. In the CI's approach, the most favourable attributes to support the development of students' competence would be openness, approachability, and the ability to have healthy interpersonal relationships and thus act as a facilitator to support students (Collier, 2018; Jayasekara et al., 2018).

One pedagogical approach to ensure that clinical teaching addresses a wide range of learning situations and the needs of a diverse population of nursing students is cognitive companionship (Deschênes et al., 2018; Lyons et al., 2017). Cognitive companionship is defined as the creation of an optimal learning environment based on social interactions for learning. The approach includes six principles that can support and guide the instructor's pedagogical actions: coaching, scaffolding, modelling, articulation, reflection, and exploration.

Coaching refers to observing students to assist and support their cognitive processes while providing specific guidance, reminders, and helpful feedback. CIs have multiple opportunities to supervise clinical judgement and reasoning in the clinical setting and to determine where students are at in the development of their competence. For example, CIs can make direct observation while students take care of patients, have students verbalize judgements and reasoning during handoffs or case presentations, and read notes that students write in the patient's chart. In all these opportunities, feedback is essential to situate students in the development of their competence. Without feedback, students can develop misconceptions, be unable to detect the seriousness of a situation, and use stereotyped or unsafe practices. In this regard, we emphasize the importance of trust, helpful interactions, and shared expectations between students and CIs.

Scaffolding refers to the support that is given to the student to achieve a level of competence that is beyond their current level. A simple way to do this is to build on the student's previous clinical experiences and knowledge while also challenging it with appropriate support. As cognitive apprentices, students actively build knowledge through their experience of authentic clinical situations. To achieve their purpose, students must encounter several examples of sufficiently similar situations in a specific domain of nursing care to develop a solid foundation of knowledge (Benner et al., 2010). For example, caring for a variety of patients in a surgical setting who have similar problems, but slightly different conditions, will help students differentiate the essential and discriminating features of their situations. The scaffolding principle can help CIs in selecting clinical situations to which students will be exposed, considering their previous clinical experiences. This allows students to exercise learning strategies such as elaboration of knowledge and comparison of key features in clinical situations, which are essential to organize and connect their knowledge library.

Regarding *modelling*, CIs are considered cognitive companions to students. As such, CIs should make their clinical judgement and reasoning visible, allowing students to model expert cognitive processes (Deschênes et al., 2021). Operationally, a CI can implement modelling by discussing a clinical situation with students, analyzing it, and indicating any conclusions they reach. At the same time, they can present their reflections, doubts, or questions that may remain unresolved as they arise. Students are thereby reassured when they realize that experts use more than one iterative phase of questioning and reflection while facing complex situations of daily practice.

Articulation involves questioning students, encouraging them to ask questions, think aloud, and verbalize their thought processes. Questioning should be used purposefully by CIs to promote clinical judgement and reasoning: "Finding the correct answer should not be perceived as the most important part of questioning; rather, the rationale underlining it should" (Merisier et al., 2018, p. 114). Students must be encouraged to ask questions to deepen their understanding of clinical situations, to articulate aloud their knowledge, and to compare their clinical judgement and reasoning processes with those of CIs or peers, highlighting similarities and differences (Deschênes et al., 2018; Deschênes et al., 2021).

Reflection consists of the retrospective examination of an experience to better understand what happened, the basis on which interventions were made, and what could have been done differently (Lavoie et al., 2017; Lavoie et al., 2013). The goal is to learn from the experience of a past clinical situation and to reinvest that learning into future experiences. Reflection allows students to review their clinical judgement and reasoning, consider the knowledge that supported them, and self-regulate by discussing with their peers and CIs and by consulting various forms of evidence, including scientific literature and evidence-based guidelines.

Exploration refers to the support provided to the student in formulating and pursuing personal learning goals, as well as assistance in helping the student find concrete ways to achieve those goals. We reiterate here the principle that competence such as clinical judgement and reasoning is developed throughout a nurse's professional life. Engaging in this philosophy of lifelong development and learning from the onset of clinical training is a pledge towards the development of expertise in nursing.

Practical Points for Effective Supervision of Clinical Judgement and Reasoning

Based on the theories and evidence presented above, we formulate some practical points to support the development of students' clinical judgement and reasoning in the clinical setting:

- Provide support appropriate to the student's level of competence. Start by being more present to coach students and then gradually decrease support. When students are more advanced, invite them to work in more challenging situations that will help them to progress and gradually gain autonomy.
- Encourage frequent articulation of knowledge, that is, encourage students to describe their thought processes aloud by organizing case discussions with you and their peers, listen to students' handoffs and follow them with feedback, and debrief after an intervention or a situation encountered in practice.
- Help students synthesize data from the situation and their knowledge into a concept map, integrating evidence to support their analysis of the situation.
- Observe how students intervene with patients (e.g., data collection, interventions) and peers (e.g., handoffs) to provide helpful hints and constructive feedback appropriate to the learning context.
- Use constructive questioning to do the following:
  - Help students identify the relevant cues in a situation and synthesize essential information (e.g., What do you notice in this situation? What is happening? What are you thinking about? What are the priorities? What supports your hypothesis? Can you summarize the situation in two to three sentences? What are your predictions about the evolution of this situation?).
  - Optimize the hypotheses generation and validation process (e.g., Have you ever experienced a similar situation? What differences or similarities have you noticed? If I remove or add this data, how would it affect your hypothesis? What are the data that confirm or refute this hypothesis? What information is missing to confirm the hypothesis? Are there other alternatives?).
  - Encourage student reflection.
- Remember that some questions trigger deeper cognitive processes than others. Try using the five Ws and one H to formulate open-ended questions: who, what, when, where, why, and how. Lower-cognitive-level questions are often closed-ended, requiring a yes or no answer (Merisier et al., 2018).
- Read students' chart notes to assess their ability to target essential data, synthesize information, and guide patient care. Clarify with the student what data are relevant and what data are missing to ensure optimal patient monitoring.
- Introduce regular debriefing sessions to analyze clinical situations encountered in the clinical setting with students. Use a reflection model to guide and structure the discussion (e.g., Lavoie et al., 2017; Lavoie et al., 2013).

- Discuss areas of ambiguity and uncertainty in clinical situations. Share your reflections and questions about the situations (Deschênes et al., 2021). This allows students to grasp your thought processes and models expert clinical judgement and reasoning.
- Invite students to analyze the development of their competence using modalities such as journaling and guided discussions to reflect, self-monitor, and self-regulate their learning and to nurture the development of their competence.
- Give regular feedback either orally or in writing. Feedback is essential to avoid the crystallization of students' difficulties and to assist in the progression of their competence (Audétat et al., 2017b, 2017c). Address difficulties promptly.

Difficulties and Remediation Strategies

Authors have highlighted the imperative for early identification of clinical judgement and reasoning difficulties in students, which can be addressed promptly to promote students' academic success (Audétat et al., 2017a; Audétat et al., 2013). Figure 4.2 presents common clinical judgement and reasoning difficulties observed in students in nursing and other health sciences (Audétat et al., 2017b, 2017c). This list is not exhaustive but may help to identify challenges and remediation strategies that CIs can implement (see Figure 4.2).

Figure 4.2 *List of Challenges and Remediation Strategies for CIs*

Difficulties	Practical remediation strategies
Difficulty in data collection	
The student has difficulty orienting data collection (i.e., data collection is either too short or too long and scattered). This difficulty frequently manifests itself in stereotypical data collection (i.e., collecting data that would be collected in any situation) without consideration of key features of the situation.	• Right after the student collects data, ask questions to help them detect relevant cues (e.g., What do you notice? What is important here? What other data should be collected? Have you encountered this situation before? How is it different?). • Verbalize your own data collection (e.g., When I see... it makes me think of... because it is similar to... and is explained by... I would like to ask... or assess...). • Prompt the student to identify relevant cues in the collected data and provide some guidance aloud (e.g., This patient's medical history indicates that frequent monitoring is required regarding...).

Difficulty in generating hypotheses	
The student fails to generate hypotheses relevant to the situation or focuses on a single hypothesis without considering alternatives (tunnel vision).	• Have the student generate two to three clinical hypotheses aloud with little information about a patient (e.g., right after handoff). • Question the student about their hypotheses (e.g., What do you think? Can you explain how you arrived at this hypothesis? What are the alternatives?). • Ask for evidence to support hypotheses and conclusions (e.g., What assessment findings support this hypothesis? Are there any contradictory findings?).
Difficulties in prioritizing	
The student does not properly prioritize interventions. This may be due to a lack of knowledge or difficulty in grasping key elements of a situation and distinguishing relevant from irrelevant data.	• Question the student about the acuity of a situation and the priority of interventions (e.g., What is important now? What makes you think this? What are the relevant facts of the situation?). • Verbalize your own understanding of the situation and prioritization of care. • Help the student anticipate how the situation might evolve (e.g., What do you think may happen in this situation?).
Difficulties in seeing the big picture	
The student fails to make connections between data related to the situation. The student focuses on isolated pieces of information without having a global vision of the situation. As a result, developing a personalized care plan is challenging.	• Ask questions to help the student synthesize relevant data (e.g., Can you summarize the situation in two to three sentences? What are the key points here?). • Listen to the student's handoffs and read their notes in the chart; follow with constructive feedback to help the student focus on the essential information to be conveyed. • Support the student in using the SBAR (situation-background-assessment-recommendation) technique to organize and synthesize their understanding of the situation.

Summary

Clinical judgement and reasoning are two sides of a nurse's clinical competence and represent an essential target of nursing education. This chapter proposed an overview of what every CI should know to support the development of students' clinical judgement and reasoning in the clinical setting. Conceptual and theoretical foundations were presented; characteristics of clinical competence were described, as well as the principles of effective supervision of clinical judgement and reasoning. Finally, practical strategies for assisting students with difficulties were identified.

CIs play a critical role in assisting students to develop sound clinical judgement and reasoning. Equipped with sufficient theoretical and evidence-based knowledge, the CI has a range of strategies to create optimal conditions for the development of students' competence in the clinical setting. Principles from the cognitive companionship approach can facilitate students' transition into the world of clinical practice. Altogether, these strategies can contribute to students' professionalization (Bélisle et al., 2021) and help them "think like a nurse" (Tanner, 2006). In addition, the cognitive companionship approach fosters the adoption of a reflective posture early in students' careers, which favours its upholding so that they become lifelong learners.

Conclusion

Nurses who begin as CIs are often experienced and seasoned. Although they have honed their clinical judgement and reasoning over time, they often struggle to clearly describe their thought processes and how they make clinical decisions, as this process is deeply embedded in who they are as clinicians. To be an excellent CI and to foster the development of students, a nurse must develop their pedagogical competence in addition to their clinical expertise. Being able to assess a student's clinical judgement and reasoning is an ability that develops over time, as is the CI's ability to make their clinical reasoning visible. Through discussion and questioning, the CI's reasoning will become more and more visible for students to learn from. If competence develops throughout a career, then every situation in the clinical setting will be a learning opportunity for the student as a nurse and the instructor as an educator.

References

Audétat, M.-C., Laurin, S., Dory, V., Charlin, B., & Nendaz, M. (2017a). Diagnosis and management of clinical reasoning difficulties: Part I. Clinical reasoning supervision and educational diagnosis. *Medical Teacher, 39*(8), 792-796. https://doi.org/10.1080/0142159X.2017.1331033

Audétat, M.-C., Laurin, S., Dory, V., Charlin, B., & Nendaz, M. (2017b). Diagnostic et prise en charge des difficultés de raisonnement clinique. Guide AMEE n° 117 (version courte)-Seconde partie: gestion des difficultés et stratégies de remédiation. *Pédagogie médicale, 18*(3), 139-149. https://doi.org/10.1051/pmed/2018011

Audétat, M.-C., Laurin, S., Dory, V., Charlin, B., & Nendaz, M. (2017c). Diagnostic et prise en charge des difficultés de raisonnement clinique. Guide AMEE no 117 (version courte)-Première partie: supervision du raisonnement clinique et diagnostic pédagogique. *Pédagogie médicale, 18*(3), 129-138. https://doi.org/10.1051/pmed/2018012

Audétat, M.-C., Laurin, S., Sanche, G., Béïque, C., Fon, N. C., Blais, J.-G., & Charlin, B. (2013). Clinical reasoning difficulties: a taxonomy for clinical teachers. *Medical Teacher, 35*(3), e984-e989. https://doi.org/10.3109/0142159X.2012.733041

Bélisle, M., Lavoie, P., Pepin, J., Fernandez, N., Boyer, L., Lechasseur, K., & Larue, C. (2021). A conceptual framework of student professionalization for health professional education and research. *International journal of nursing education scholarship, 18*(1), 20200104. https://doi.org/10.1515/ijnes-2020-0104

Benner, P. (1984). *From novice to expert: Excellence and power in clinical practice*. Addison-Wesley.

Benner, P., Sutphen, M., Leonard, V., & Day, L. (2010). *Educating nurses: A call for radical transformation*. Jossey-Bass.

Boyer, L., Tardif, J., & Lefebvre, H. (2015). From a medical problem to a health experience: How nursing students think in clinical situations. *Journal of Nursing Education, 54*(11), 625-632. https://doi.org/10.3928/01484834-20151016-03

Charette, M., McKenna, L. G., Deschênes, M.-F., Ha, L., Merisier, S., & Lavoie, P. (2020). New graduate nurses' clinical competence: A mixed methods systematic review. *Journal of Advanced Nursing, 76*(11), 2810-2829. https://doi.org/10.1111/jan.14487

Collier, A. D. (2018). Characteristics of an effective nursing clinical instructor: The state of the science. *Journal of Clinical Nursing, 27*(1-2), 363-374. https://doi.org/10.1111/jocn.13931

Deschênes, M.-F., Boyer, L., Fernandez, N., & Goudreau, J. (2018). Le compagnonnage cognitif: une approche pédagogique à explorer pour le développement du raisonnement clinique infirmier ? *Quality Advancement in Nursing Education-Avancées en formation infirmière, 4*(2), Article 5, 1-17. https://doi.org/10.17483/2368-6669.1156

Deschênes, M.-F., Létourneau, D., & Goudreau, J. (2021). Script concordance approach in nursing education. *Nurse Educator*. https://doi.org/10.1097/NNE.0000000000001028

Evans, J. S., & Stanovich, K. E. (2013). Dual-process theories of higher cognition: Advancing the debate. *Perspectives on Psychological Science, 8*(3), 223-241. https://doi.org/10.1177/1745691612460685

Jarvis, C. (2018). *Physical examination and health assessment – Canadian e-book*. Elsevier Health Sciences.

Jayasekara, R., Smith, C., Hall, C., Rankin, E., Smith, M., Visvanathan, V., & Friebe, T.-R. (2018). The effectiveness of clinical education models for undergraduate nursing programs: A systematic review. *Nurse Education in Practice, 29*, 116-126. https://doi.org/10.1016/j.nepr.2017.12.006

Lavoie, P., Boyer, L., Pepin, J. I., Goudreau, J., & Fima, O. (2017). Accompagner les infirmières et les étudiantes dans la réflexion sur des situations de soins : Un modèle pour les formateurs en soins infirmiers. *Quality Advancement in Nursing Education – Avancées en formation infirmière*, 3(1). https://doi.org/10.17483/2368-6669.1100

Lavoie, P., Pepin, J., & Boyer, L. (2013). Reflective debriefing to promote novice nurses' clinical judgment after high-fidelity clinical simulation: A pilot test. *Dynamics*, 24(4), 36–41.

Lyons, K., McLaughlin, J. E., Khanova, J., & Roth, M. (2017). Cognitive apprenticeship in health sciences education: a qualitative review. *Advances in Health Sciences Education*, 22(3), 723–739. https://doi.org/10.1007/s10459-016-9707-4

Melin-Johastudentson, C., Palmqvist, R., & Ronnberg, L. (2017). Clinical intuition in the nursing process and decision-making-A mixed-studies review. *Journal of Clinical Nursing*, 26(23–24), 3936–3949. https://doi.org/10.1111/jocn.13814

Merisier, S., Larue, C., & Boyer, L. (2018). How does questioning influence nursing students' clinical reasoning in problem-based learning? A scoping review. *Nurse Education Today*, 65, 108–115. https://doi.org/10.1016/j.nedt.2018.03.006

Monteiro, S., Sherbino, J., Sibbald, M., & Norman, G. (2020). Critical thinking, biases and dual processing: The enduring myth of generalisable skills. *Medical Education*, 54(1), 66–73. https://doi.org/10.1111/medu.13872

Simpson, E., & Courtney, M. (2002). Critical thinking in nursing education: Literature review. *International Journal of Nursing Practice*, 8(2), 89–98. https://doi.org/10.1046/j.1440-172x.2002.00340.x

Tanner, C. A. (2006). Thinking like a nurse: A research-based model of clinical judgment in nursing. *Journal of Nursing Education*, 45, 204–211. https://doi.org/10.3928/01484834-20060601-04

Tiffen, J., Corbridge, S. J., & Slimmer, L. (2014). Enhancing clinical decision making: Development of a contiguous definition and conceptual framework. *Journal of Professional Nursing*, 30(5), 399–405. https://doi.org/10.1016/j.profnurs.2014.01.006

CHAPTER 5

Practice-Based Learning in Acute Care Settings

Kariane Holmes

This chapter takes a deeper look into the role of the clinical instructor when supporting nursing students in acute care placement settings. Using the principles of practice-based learning, creative and practical strategies in the form of clinical learning activities are integrated for new clinical instructors to creatively support nursing students through a process of learner reflexivity across all stages of the acute care clinical practicum.

Chapter Objectives

After completing the chapter, the reader will be able to
- outline a successful orientation that prepares nursing students and the acute placement unit for a collaborative learning experience
- describe the competencies and understand the expectations of nursing students in acute clinical practicums
- develop appropriate patient assignments for nursing students at varying learner abilities
- outline how to lead successful pre- and post-clinical conferences
- explain how to support nursing students through unexpected clinical encounters or challenges that may present in acute care clinical practicums
- illustrate how to successfully evaluate and provide feedback in a timely fashion to both nursing students and precepting staff nurses in a manner that motivates ongoing learning

Introduction

Clinical practicums are often an exciting time and one of the most anticipated aspects of pre-service education for nursing students (Mirlashari et al., 2017). Acute care placements offer practice-based learning opportunities, bringing to life theoretical concepts acquired in the classroom through real and meaningful patient encounters. For some students, this transition can also bring challenges that interfere with their ability to acquire new experiential knowledge and skills, particularly in difficult situations in an acute care placement setting (Lundberg, 2008). Clinical instructors (CIs) must be supportive and prepared to manage these challenges at all phases of the acute clinical practicum to ensure that the benefits of practice-based learning are maximized as they educate and motivate the upcoming generation of nursing professionals.

Background and History of Acute Care Placement Settings

In Chapter 2, the adaptation of the CI role was explored as nursing education transitioned from hospital to academia. During this transition, educators recognized the need for integrative practice-based experiences, especially towards the end of baccalaureate nursing programs (Canadian Association of Schools of Nursing [CASN], 2012). The first integrated nursing program was introduced at the University of Toronto in 1942 (CASN, 2012). Today, students still fulfil academic requirements by completing theory-based courses at colleges and universities, augmented by hospital-based clinical courses (CASN, 2012).

Since the early 20th century, teaching philosophies have evolved from telling nursing students *what* they needed to know to work in acute settings to teaching them *how* to practise in a broad range of areas (Kozier et al., 2014). CIs have adopted a pedagogical approach that encourages nursing students to think critically and use the best available science-based evidence when providing care (Kozier et al., 2014; Registered Nurses' Association of Ontario [RNAO], (2016). This conceptualized tactic is especially important in acute practice areas, which are often fast-paced and cover a range of specialized knowledge and competencies.

Large teaching hospitals have traditionally been the primary setting for nursing student placements (Smith et al., 2013; van Iersel et al., 2020). Clinical placements can be adapted to accommodate a group with larger nursing student-to-CI ratios or a single student with a one-nursing-student-to-preceptor approach. The former often occurs during the earlier years of pre-service nursing education, with the latter in the next to last or final semester. These placements are aimed at providing real-time learning opportunities facilitated by CIs in a variety of settings that will reflect nursing students' experiences after graduation.

According to the Canadian Institutes of Health Research (CIHR), nurses in hospital care settings account for 65.57% of nurses across Canada, versus community and long-term-care settings (CIHR, 2019). Further data show that about half of new graduate nurses practise on medical-surgical units or on other specialized units, including critical care, obstetrics, or pediatrics (Spence Laschinger et al., 2019). Educational programs must equip nursing students with the knowledge, attitudes, and skills that they will need as new graduate nurses to provide safe and effective care in these acute care specialities (Kozier et al., 2014).

In a national survey of clinical placement settings for students across Canada by Smith et al. (2013), all but three hospitals reported using medical-surgical inpatient units as a component of acute practice placement requirements. Acute medical-surgical units are often viewed as relevant and desirable placements, accepting students from a variety of different health care programs. This high volume of students can make it difficult for staff to consistently provide individualized support. It is the responsibility of CIs to help nursing students navigate opportunities in acute placement settings to ensure a meaningful practice-based application of knowledge and preparation for entry-to-nursing practice.

Setting the Stage

Orientation

CIs set the stage for a positive learning experience and motivation through orientation activities (CASN, 2012). Attention to careful preparation serves as an example for students to follow and role models how to prepare effectively for clinical shifts. Students report having to be ready to work as soon as they start acute care placements (Morley et al., 2015). Setting the stage with an organized orientation that provides adequate time for students to arrive and settle into an acute care setting is essential for cultivating an inviting learning environment (MacDonald et al., 2016).

The academic institution or clinical practice facility will often have a checklist of activities that the CI must complete during the clinical orientation process. However, these checklists are often not unit or hospital specific. Students may also need to complete learning modules and certifications and fulfil health and safety requirements specific to the clinical practice environment before their arrival. The CI must ensure that each of these components is completed and provide a thorough orientation as they introduce students to the clinical practice environment.

Nursing students have found that receiving written information before arriving at their in-person orientation helped in their preparation for acute placement settings (MacDonald et al., 2016). This tangible package is a valuable learning tool that helps students absorb the often-overwhelming volume of information they receive when they first arrive at the clinical placement (MacDonald et al., 2016). Chapter 2 discussed the possibility of CIs generating a website to connect with students and share this information before their arrival. CIs should investigate to see what information students have already received from the academic facility and what orientation material is available from the clinical placement setting. They can then add any additional information pertinent to the acute placement setting that would be useful for students to know beforehand. A list of some materials CIs could choose to include in an information package is detailed in Figure 5.1.

Figure 5.1 *List of Materials to Be Included in a Student Nurse Orientation Package*

- Glossary of important terms related to the acute placement specialty
- Schedule of the orientation day and where to meet the CI
- Layout of a daily schedule and shift patterns (time to arrive on the unit, nursing handover, initial assessment, routine care and vital sign frequency, standard medication times, breaks, etc.)
- Location of key areas that will be toured on the "wayfinding" component of the in-person orientation (e.g., change rooms, washrooms, cafeteria, parking)
- Key contact information (include your information as the CI and that of any other key members of the clinical practice team or academic institution)
- Dress code and items to include in a clinical bag (pens, ID badge, calculator, watch, stethoscope, notepad, change of clothes)
- Professional conduct expectations
- Assignment due dates

- Acute placement emergency codes and the nursing student's expected response
- Important phone numbers and who to call in an emergency or illness
- Frequently asked questions
- Possibly common diagnosis, medications, and procedures

Source: Adapted from a clinical learning activity in MacDonald et al. (2016).

To ensure a successful welcoming orientation when students arrive at the clinical practice setting, CIs should have uninterrupted and dedicated time to complete the orientation process before having students provide patient care. There should be adequate time for students to complete most, if not all, activities (i.e., wayfinding, scavenger hunt), ask questions, and share concerns with the CI before interacting with patients and the unit staff.

Wayfinding

Wayfinding is the initial exposure whereby students are introduced to the clinical environment and to potential learning experiences (Worrall, 2007). Students have reported that a tour of the unit in which important rooms and equipment are identified contributes to their feeling a sense of belonging in their clinical practice placement (Worrall, 2007). These unit-specific items may include, but are not limited to, where to find physicians' orders, medication administration records, medication room, equipment room, clean and dirty storage, linens, isolation rooms, and procedure carts. Other key areas that should be included on a wayfinding tour of the hospital include staff washrooms, breakrooms, locker or changing rooms, cafeteria, parking areas, visitor waiting areas, diagnostic imaging areas, manager's office, and the hospital library or other locations where students can find resources such as reference guides and relevant journals.

Clinical Learning Activity: Scavenger Hunt

Scavenger hunts are a fun learner-centred activity that builds on the wayfinding aspect of orientation. This learning activity sets the groundwork for reflexive learning as students become immersed in the placement setting by exploring, engaging with, and experiencing their new clinical environment (Afolayan, 2016). The goal of a scavenger hunt is for students to feel empowered to provide care or assistance by building their confidence as they navigate the unit and locate supplies they will use either during acute situations or for routine daily practices.

A scavenger hunt is made up of two phases: (1) a clue is provided by the CI and (2) the student locates that item and either returns it to the CI or provides an answer related to the clue. The clues provided by the CI can range in difficulty and be adapted to a learner's critical thinking ability, rooted in the principles of learner reflexivity. The following examples of locating a blood glucose monitor demonstrate a range of clues that engage students in a range of critical thinking concepts, increasing in difficulty as they become more involved in the acute placement setting:

- Remember: "Find the blood glucose monitor."
- Understand: "Identify the tool that you must use before administering insulin."
- Apply: "Locate a piece of equipment that can help you interpret your patient's symptoms of tachycardia, irritability, dizziness, sweating, shakiness, diaphoresis while they are NPO."

Alternatively, if CIs are unfamiliar with creating their own scavenger hunt, a great starting place is to use common policies or procedures on the unit and have students locate the equipment that will be needed to perform a specific skill. Using the example above, CIs can use the policy or patient care plan on managing hypoglycemia. Not only will students be navigating the process of accessing a policy, but they will also be able to conceptualize the meaning of procedure and locate the supplies required to carry out the tasks in the scavenger hunt.

Shadow Shift

The remainder of the dedicated orientation time may be spent by observing or "shadowing" one of the staff nurses on the unit. Shadow shifts may also serve as a transition period between the orientation time and the clinical placement shift. CIs must be clear with students and unit staff that the purpose of the shadow shift is not to perform patient care or to begin demonstrating competencies; rather it is part of the orientation process to become acquainted with the nurse's workflow and the layout of the clinical practice setting. MacDonald et al. (2016) found that students who had a complete orientation on their first shift in a clinical setting felt more at ease with their surroundings and with the nursing process. Further, when staff nurses invited students to join them for a shadow shift, the nurses found they were less rushed during particularly busy times (such as at the beginning of a shift following handover), and they appreciated having more time to spend orienting their students (MacDonald et al., 2016).

Managing External Factors

External factors that students bring to the acute placement setting can impact their clinical learning experience and level of preparation. These factors include managing household duties, balancing academic workloads, and experiencing fatigue and loneliness (MacDonald et al., 2016). It is imperative for the CI to share with the academic and clinical practice staff, without naming students, some of the challenges that students encounter before and during the clinical practicum. By understanding these external factors, CIs can help students manage challenges so that they can optimize their learning, be present, and learn through real-time clinical experiences (MacDonald et al., 2019). CIs should be aware of available services, such as clinical counselling or academic advisers in the academic institution, and direct students to them if the CIs are unable to help students address challenging external factors.

Travel to the Placement

Travel is a common feature of clinical placements (Smith et al., 2013). Most students report needing to do at least some commuting to their clinical placement setting (Smith et al., 2013). Clinical placements in some acute practice settings can occur between 7 a.m. and 11 p.m., in 8- or 12-hour day or evening shifts (University of Alberta, 2021). After students have arranged their transportation according to their clinical placement schedule, CIs can ease students' commuting transition and adjustment to shiftwork by having a structured pre-conference time. Structured pre-conference times can help students plan both their time to travel to their placement and the time they will spend there. For more details on pre-conferences, see section *Foundations of Acute Care Setting Practicums*.

Expectations of the Acute Care Practicum: Understanding Limitations

The Canadian Nurses Association (CNA, 2015, p. 30) outlines examples of regulatory body entry-level registered nurse (RN) competency statements. CIs can use the CNA (2015) *Framework for the Practice of Registered Nurses in Canada* to prepare nursing students for practice in acute care placement settings. The CI should emphasize that nursing student autonomy in acute placements settings can be limited because of the complexity of patient care needs and that students may need additional training to perform certain tasks or care for acute-level patients (Gonzalez-Garcia et al., 2020).

CIs set this expectation early to minimize students' disappointment or frustration with a perceived lack of technical skill development. This is especially important if students have experienced enhanced autonomy in previous clinical placement rotations. For more details on a clinical teaching strategy to help students understanding their limitations, see the section Clinical Learning Activity: Badge Attachment of Do's and Don'ts later in this chapter and the section Working with Pre-service Professionals.

During the orientation period, CIs may suggest learning outcomes for students as they begin to set goals for their learning plan or accompanying academic work. This guidance helps students identify experiences they might not have realized were available in the acute placement setting (Worrall, 2007). CIs can also help nursing students identify these potential learning outcomes during the clinical pre-conference by focusing on realistic day-to-day expectations and short-term learning goals.

Access to Charting and Patient Information

Ensuring that students are familiar with the charting system, and ways of gathering patient information, can effectively enhance their clinical learning experiences and should be an essential component of the orientation. Although as a CI you may already be familiar with accessing patient information, consider what this process may seem like to a student new to the acute placement setting (Melrose et al., 2015). Melrose et al. (2015) suggest making a list of various communication, charting, and information-gathering tools used in your clinical placement area and comparing these to other tools that students have learned about either in a simulation lab or during a classroom theory course.

Nursing students often work across various practice facilities as they rotate through clinical placement settings and will be introduced to several charting and information-gathering systems (Melrose et al., 2015). Whether students are using a paper-based charting system or a new online interface, the way in which they gather and document patient information and the amount can be overwhelming. CIs need to understand documentation and communication procedures specific to each placement facility. For example, CIs need to know how students can access patient data, whether they require passwords, and whether they need to complete specific training modules (Melrose et al., 2015). Other considerations include knowing what students can and cannot document and what information they can or cannot access as these systems are considered legal documents.

Students should have access to charting and patient information systems in a timely manner, ideally before they arrive on the clinical unit. CIs can use dedicated time during pre- or post-clinical conferences, or during a clinical lab, to orient students to relevant communication and documentation tools so that these activities do not consume their practice experience time (Melrose et al., 2015).

Clinical Learning Activity: Seek and Find a Patient Chart

Similar to the Clinical Learning Activity: Scavenger Hunt, the purpose is to enhance nursing student proficiency in accessing patient information before providing care. CIs can encourage students either individually or in pairs to choose a patient chart and identify the details necessary for selecting a patient assignment. This activity also orients students to the expected charting and documentation requirements of the acute placement setting. The following prompts for this clinical learning activity are adapted from the CASN Clinical Instructor Nurse Educator Interest Group (2015):

- Physician or doctor's order sheet: What are the most current and up to date orders? Are there any orders outstanding?
- Nursing narrative notes or patient progress record: What type of charting is completed on a daily basis? Monthly? Hourly?
- Admission history: When and why was this patient admitted to the unit?
- Admission assessment: Was an activities of daily living assessment included?
- List of conditions: How would you determine the conditions that are a priority for this patient? Current concerns versus those that are no longer a problem?
- Discharge planning: How do you find information when this patient is scheduled to be discharged from the unit? What remains outstanding before their discharge?
- Medication list: When are the standard medication times?
- Do not resuscitate orders and advance directives

Fitting In and Unit Culture

The acute placement setting offers students the opportunity to begin their professional socialization into the nursing culture (Gilbert & Brown, 2015). A sense of belonging, acceptance, and affirmation from staff and patients have been identified as highly important to students in a quality clinical learning experience (Courtney-Pratt et al., 2011; Gilbert & Brown, 2015). Nursing students who do not feel a sense of belonging and fitting in with the unit culture can experience decreased motivation to learn in their clinical rotation (Worrall, 2007). Therefore, ensuring that students are accepted as valuable contributing members of the unit team will enhance their eagerness to learn, increase their resilience in acute care scenarios, and facilitate a positive learning experience that will influence their success in future practice.

Positive professional socialization experiences can benefit safe patient care. Students reported increased confidence to seek advice and ask for help with their patient care when they experienced positive and accepting relationships with their precepting nurses (Courtney-Pratt et al., 2011). Consequences of a dysfunctional unit culture may include students feeling anxious, nervous, and incompetent, and a perceived lack of motivation by the preceptors will further perpetuate a deficient learning culture (Courtney-Pratt et al., 2011). CIs can ensure a successful beginning to this professional socialization process by focusing on getting acquainted with their students before the clinical placement starts. When CIs know their students, they are better able to introduce them successfully to the nurses and staff on the placement unit. CIs should also take care to support the precepting nurses to help foster positive relationships between the students and preceptors. Further, CIs are responsible for cultivating a positive relationship with others who work on the unit that is hosting the students. Being pleasant, approachable, respectful, and helpful are important skills for CIs who are nurturing these positive relationships.

Getting to Know Your Students

The CASN (2015) recommends that before starting each clinical placement rotation, CIs should arrange private one-on-one meetings with each student. These meetings can occur in person or online using the university's approved platform. Inviting students to this instructor-student relationship develops a greater sense of connection and can enhance the learning process. These meetings help CIs identify the best strategies for supporting the individual learning needs of each nursing student. Doing so can facilitate the delivery of safe care to the patients in the acute placement setting (CASN, 2015). CASN (2015) provides suggested questions for this first meeting with students (see Box 5.1).

Box 5.1 *Questions CIs Should Ask During the First Meeting with Students*

- What are your preferred name and pronouns?
- What is your preferred and fastest method for contact and confirmations (email, phone)?
- What is your preferred style of learning? Can you give an example?
- What are some personal strengths and challenges from previous clinical placements (if any)?
- How can I best support you as a learner?
- What do you expect from me?
- What are you most excited about in this clinical placement?
- What are you most worried about?
- What are your career goals as an RN?
- Do you have any nurses in your family or experience in health care?
- Do you work outside school?
- What do you like to do in your free time?
- Are there any other concerns or information that you would like to share?

Source: Based on CASN (2015).

Knowing your students on a more personal level, and understanding their professional aspirations, will help students feel comfortable in reaching out to you as the CI during the placement. It may also help the CI when developing patient assignments, setting goals, and personalizing evaluation methods. Your knowledge of students may help if students ask you to act as a reference when they apply for new graduate nursing positions. Finally, this set of questions provides a non-threatening way for students to express any concerns regarding the acute care placement setting that they may not feel comfortable sharing in person or in a group setting.

Addressing Student Concerns, Fears, and Anxieties

CIs must recognize that the abundance of information provided to students during the orientation process can overwhelm students and may increase stress rather than alleviate previous fears or concerns (Worrall, 2007). Failure to acknowledge this can contribute to students concerns, fears, and anxieties, and prevent them from experiencing effective growth and learning in the acute placement setting (Jamshidi et al., 2016). Ensuring students receive the support they need to succeed in clinical placements is essential. In the most serious of situations, students have left the profession as a direct result of unresolved fear and anxiety experienced during clinical placements in acute care settings.

In the orientation package, it was suggested that CIs include a section of frequently asked questions (FAQs) related to the acute clinical placement setting. CIs can modify this list for each clinical group, asking for input from students about what they would have found useful as they prepared for the clinical placement. CIs can use this input as a guide to address specific student concerns, help ease their transition, and minimize student concerns and anxieties in preparation for the acute care placement practicum.

CIs need to give students permission and encourage them to ask questions and ask others on the unit for assistance if needed. Al Shahrani (2015) found that students were better able to cope with the stressors of their first clinical placement when they asked the CI or staff nurses clarifying questions. This was especially important when questions pertained to nursing skills students felt inadequately prepared to perform confidently. Asking for help to perform such skills should be emphasized as a strength for students as it indicates that they are concerned about providing optimum care and avoiding negative patient outcomes. Students need to know that asking for assistance when needed is not an indicator of incompetence (Al Shahrani, 2015). In fact, CIs should be concerned if they notice that students stop asking questions. When CIs encourage students to ask questions and for assistance, they are ensuring patient safety while simultaneously supporting students becoming part of the care team. CIs should emphasize the value of team collaboration when practising as a nursing student and as an experienced nurse in the acute clinical setting.

Interprofessional Collaboration

Interprofessional collaboration is defined by the Canadian Interprofessional Health Collaborative (CIHC, 2010) as "a partnership between a team of health providers and a client in a participatory, collaborative and coordinated approach to shared decision-making around health and social issues" (p. 11). Academic institutions negotiate clinical placements with health care facilities that host acute care clinical practicums for students. The success of these placements is based on the mutual respect for professional values in the service delivery to patients and a professional commitment to the future nursing generation (Courtney-Pratt et al., 2011). Therefore, students are not exempt from the CIHC (2010) relational efforts when in the acute care clinical setting as they work with members of the health care team to provide patient care.

CIs are pivotal in facilitating the integration of students into the interprofessional team throughout their clinical experience. When students learn how to function as interprofessional team members during clinical placements, it prepares them for these interactions post-graduation. This integration into the clinical learning environment enhances students' sense of belonging and fitting into the unit culture (Gilbert & Brown, 2015). A scoping literature review by Murdoch et al. (2017) found that the use of various interprofessional frameworks and learning activities promotes interprofessional collaboration in the humanistic and dynamic context of the acute care placement setting. These frameworks and activities equip students to become new graduate nurses with the knowledge, communication skills, and attitudes to participate as effective members of the health care team (Murdoch et al., 2017).

The interprofessional experience should begin with early exposure in the practice environment, such as with an introduction session for students where they meet key members of the unit staff (Murdoch et al., 2017; Worrall, 2007). These introductions can be included in the orientation day and have been demonstrated to help students feel a sense of belonging in the practice environment (Worrall, 2007). Some of these key members students should meet may include, but are not limited to, the charge nurse, nursing manager, nursing educator, unit lead staff physician, and unit clerk. Other opportunities for students to engage with members of the interprofessional team include organizing brief talks or "lunch and learns" during post-conference where a team member provides an informal overview of their role. This integration and relationship building outside the clinical practice time will enhance nursing student confidence to work with various members of the interprofessional team in the acute care placement setting.

Professional Conduct

Acute placement settings may be students' first introduction to the practice environment. Regardless of experience in the clinical placement environment, students are held to the same professional conduct standards as any other health care professional. CIs must inform and enforce the professional standards of practice and have non-negotiable consequences for breaches of professional conduct. CIs must be familiar with the code of conduct and professional standards from the clinical setting organization, regulating nursing body, and academic institution.

One of the most important aspects of professional conduct in the acute placement setting is ensuring confidentiality and the privacy of the patients and their families. Students are often excited and eager to share their learning experiences with others outside the circle of care. However, CIs must convey to students that such breaches can have long-term negative consequences that may impact their future nursing career or have legal consequences. CIs should provide examples of breaches and ways that students can share their learnings without violating patient privacy or confidentiality. For more information on professional conduct and ethical and legal standards for CIs in the acute placement setting refer to Chapter 8.

Foundations of Acute Care Setting Practicums

Understanding Curriculum and Unit-Specific Policies

CIs are the intersection for students as they integrate policies and resources of the placement setting with the curriculum of the academic institution. As mentioned previously, CIs need to have realistic expectations regarding what learning outcomes students can achieve in the acute placement setting. The following is a guide for CIs to help them support students as pre-service professionals to ensure that they are fulfilling the learning outcomes within their defined scope of practice.

Pre-conference

Pre-conference is a purposeful yet brief meeting between the CI and students that precedes clinical learning activities at the start of a shift (Gaberson & Oermann, 1999; Wink, 1995). These meetings are student-centred and can occur as a one-to-one meeting, or in a clinical small group setting in a protected environment (Gaberson & Oermann, 1999; Health Alliance of MidAmerica LLC, n.d.). Pre-clinical conferences were first described by Matheney (1969) as a time for students to receive their assignments, review patient information and records, set care goals, develop a plan of care, and ask questions or express concerns regarding their upcoming clinical shift.

Pre-conferences should be short and focus on what students will be completing throughout upcoming clinical shift (Health Alliance of MidAmerica LLC, n.d.). These meetings are also an opportunity for CIs to assess and validate the student's level of preparation specific to their patient assignment if the assignment was received the night before the shift (Health Alliance of MidAmerica LLC, n.d.). CIs can assess student preparedness and ensure patient safety by asking critical thinking questions, such as "What are your top three priorities for this patient today?" (Bristol, 2021). Pre-conferences can also serve as a time for CIs to review students' daily expectations and to help students organize their day (see the activity later in this chapter titled Clinical Learning Activity: Day Planners, Time Sheets, and a Nurse's Brain). Pre-conference meetings are an important opportunity for helping students develop critical thinking skills. CIs and students engage in conversation whereby the CI may ask questions that help students make connections between theory and their upcoming clinical practice activities, anticipate actions, and determine a focus for patient assessments (Health Alliance of MidAmerica LLC, n.d.).

Finally, pre-conferences offer an opportunity for CIs to address any student concerns or stressors and to discuss any values and assumptions that will influence care delivery (Wink, 1995). Pre-conferences can be used to manage students concerns, helping to ensure a focused, grounded, and optimistic beginning for a clinical learning experience.

Developing Patient Assignments

Developing patient assignments to advance the knowledge of students was first described in 1945 by registered nurse Helen F. Nicholson. Nicholson (1945) valued this important task of the head nurse, or in the academic setting, the CI. Nicholson emphasized that "assignments are planned to provide the greatest possible learning opportunities for students which will in turn result in better nursing care for patients" (p. 1055). CIs should thoughtfully arrange student patient assignments before students arrive in the acute placement setting (Akuamoah-Boateng, n.d.). The patient assignment process should be made in collaboration with a leadership representative for the unit (i.e., a charge nurse or unit manager), with the goal of fulfilling the needs of both the organization staff and the learners (Akuamoah-Boateng, n.d.).

There is debate between leaders in academic facilities and administrators in acute placement settings as to whether students should be privy to information regarding their assigned patients before their clinical shift. CIs should familiarize themselves with the practice and expectations of their faculty and placement setting before students' first clinical shift and inform students of when they can expect to be notified about their patient assignments. The timing of the notification will determine expectations regarding preparation for clinical shifts. If patient assignment details are provided to students before they arrive at their clinical shifts, this should occur no more than 24 hours in advanced as the status of patients changes quickly in acute settings. Students should be provided with information that includes medical diagnoses, conditions, diagnostic tests, and medications (Herdman, 2012).

The number of patients and workload should be assigned based on each student's scope of practice and learning goals, and the current needs of the unit. For the first patient assignment, students should be assigned only one patient. Nursing students must demonstrate their ability to manage and safely care for one patient in an acute placement setting before their level of responsibility is increased by adding additional patients to their workload. CIs should understand how many patients students are expected to care for as the term progresses. For example, the faculty may require that students care for two or three patients by the end of the semester if they are further along in their pre-service education program. In this case, CIs can incrementally increase the patient workload as they assess the student is safely able to do so.

Alternatively, some institutions request that students determine their own clinical assignments rather than being assigned patients by the CI. Self-selection of patients benefits students as they become more self-directed and have increased confidence, autonomy, and motivation when making patient selections (Montgomery, 2009). Students report that the self-selection process allows them to choose an assignment that meets their individual learning needs and provides an opportunity to evaluate their own learning more effectively (Montgomery, 2009).

Before CIs can invite students to self-select patients, students should be proficient in accessing patient information. The Clinical Learning Activity: Seek and Find a Patient Chart described earlier in the chapter builds on the Clinical Learning Activity: Scavenger Hunt and can be used to facilitate the process as students prepare to self-select their patient assignments. CIs need to review the student-selected assignments before starting the clinical shift to ensure the assignments are appropriateness in relation to students' learning needs and course objectives, and the needs of the host facility (Montgomery, 2009).

It should be made clear to all health care providers that students are supernumerary to the nurses responsible for the patients the students are caring for. CIs should inform staff at the beginning of each shift about the clinical objectives and scope of practice, and what they can expect from of the students during their time on the unit (Akuamoah-Boateng, n.d.). See the Clinical Learning Activity: Badge Attachment of Do's and Dont's later in the chapter for an accessible way to communicate this information to staff nurses and students. If the communication of expectations is clear, students and supervising nurses can collaborate to generate a plan for the upcoming shift. The CI can act as a liaison to help facilitate this collaborative process.

To avoid overwhelming staff nurses who are taking on additional responsibility by mentoring student nurses, CIs should do their best to assign only one student to a nurse on the unit and not to assign a student to a nurse who is also precepting a new graduate or new hire (Akuamoah-Boateng, n.d.). Optimal pairing of students with staff nurses is instrumental in creating a positive and motivating learning experience and professional socialization, especially in highly acute clinical placement settings.

Preparing for Patient Assignments

If students receive patient information before their arrival on the unit, CIs should guide students to focus on what they need to know to care for their assigned patient beforehand as they work towards developing a care plan rather than planning and anticipating a task-based plan of care (Herdman, 2012). For example, students should have a foundational understanding of the overarching concepts and nursing considerations when caring for a patient with congestive heart failure (i.e., diuresis) versus knowing the timing of a patient's daily dose of furosemide. What tasks students actually need to do will be discovered upon arrival at the unit as orders often change, especially in acute placement settings. Also, focusing on overarching concepts supports the development of clinical reasoning and higher-level thinking (Herdman, 2012). Using the example of diuresis and a patient with congestive heart failure, the nursing student will discover the timing of the furosemide dose upon arrival at the unit, when reviewing the medical administration record. From their preparatory work, students should then consider the patient's recent lab values, including electrolytes, before administering medication. They should also have already completed a cardiorespiratory assessment, including fluid balance, that they will reassess after administering the medication. As this example demonstrates, having a foundational knowledge of pathophysiology and pharmacology and related higher-level nursing concepts allows students to concentrate on anticipatory nursing actions that may guide their focused assessment and development of nursing care plans.

Working with Pre-service Professionals

Students are considered pre-service learners in the registered nursing profession. RNs have a scope that is defined by their employment or academic institution based on their level of education (College of Registered Nurses of Manitoba [CRNM], 2018). Students are accountable to the academic institution, clinical placement setting, and ultimately government regulation of the Act governing the health professions in the licensing jurisdiction (CRNM, 2018; University of British Columbia [UBC], 2016). The CI must be familiar with scope of practice of students within each of these. For example, UBC (2016, p. 3) has developed a hierarchy-based figure used to describe the four levels of RN scope of practice, with an additional two levels for pre-service learners.

Further, CIs should familiarize themselves with (and share with their students) the difference between activities that are not restricted, such as assisting a patient with activities of daily living; restricted activities that require an order, including medication administration; and activities that are outside their scope of practice and must be delegated to a more experienced health care professional (UBC, 2016). See the Clinical Learning Activity: Badge Attachment of Do's and Don'ts for further details on clinical skills that can guide CIs and students in the decision-making process regarding scope. Although this process works for task-based competencies in the acute placement setting, CIs should balance students' task-based skill acquisition with their ongoing development of skills in synthesizing nursing knowledge for a particular patient to solve problems, critically reflect, and integrate evidence-based evidence into care (Ironside et al., 2014).

Clinical Learning Activity: Badge Attachment of Do's and Don'ts

A small reference sheet of do's and don'ts can be attached to the back of an ID badge (or fit in a small pocket). This can be provided to students and nurses who will be supervising and working with nursing students. Having a small accessible reference page for students, staff nurses, and the CI will help when discerning what students can and cannot do in the acute placement setting. Green activities (do's) indicate activities that are unrestricted and nursing students can complete independently, providing they have the individual level of competence. Examples of a green activity would be assisting in activities of daily living. Yellow activities are considered conditional activities that students may perform under supervision of a qualified individual, such as the assigned staff nurse or the CI (UBC, 2016). Students must be deemed competent, even if supervised, to perform yellow activities (UBC, 2016). An example of a yellow activity is medication administration via the intravenous route. Finally, red activities (don'ts) are those that nursing students are not permitted to perform (UBC, 2016). For example, nursing students must not perform an intubation, even in code situations, as this is not within the nursing student or RN scope of practice.

During their orientation, CIs are encouraged to ask for or create a list of common activities and skills that are performed on the acute placement unit. This list can be useful for creating the badge attachment. Because of the complexity and number of skills nurses perform on acute care units, many sites already have a list of nursing student's do's and don'ts. CIs should actively seek this resource and share it with their students. Some acute placement settings require a specialized or additional certification to perform certain skills, such as the administration of chemotherapy. Students are not permitted to perform these certifiable skills. CIs should also be familiar with these specialized skills specific to their acute placements setting. Even though students may not be permitted to perform these certifiable skills, CIs should facilitate student observation of an RN performing these skills to enhance the learning opportunities for students.

A template example, true to size, of a nursing student do's and don'ts badge attachment is provided in Figure 5.2. CIs can copy this badge attachment and fill it in based on the scope of practice guidelines of students in their jurisdiction, academic institution, and acute placement facilities.

Badge attachments or pocket-sized pages are great way for CIs to consolidate other pertinent and essential information for the acute placement setting. Other information that CIs can put on a badge clip include the rights of medication administration, vital sign parameters for various age groups, and so on.

Figure 5.2 *Nursing Student Do's and Don'ts*

GREEN	YELLOW	RED
Skills or activities that nursing students may perform independently	Skills that nursing students may perform, if assessed as competent AND supervised by a qualified individual	Skills that nursing students MUST NOT perform under any circumstances

A Day in the Life: Creating an Organized Routine

CIs should arrive at the unit early, before the nursing students, to inform staff nurses that students will be on the floor for that day. Even though the charge nurse or nursing leaders may be aware of the arrival of the clinical group, individual nurses may be learning this information as they receive their patient assignments. Just as students like to be prepared for their shifts, it is important to extend this transparency and preparedness courtesy to staff nurses who will be supervising students. This early arrival also offers you as the CI an opportunity to review or modify the students' patient assignments. Please see the section Developing Patient Assignments earlier in the chapter. CIs should also ensure dedicated meeting space is booked before students arrive for clinical so that the start is not rushed and does not take away from the protected time of pre- or post-conference.

For students, a typical day shift at the clinical placement may look like the one outlined in Figure 5.3. CIs can use this organized routine as a structure for developing their own timeline to send out students ahead of their clinical placement. Additionally, CIs should review the routine times and tasks as part of the orientation process. It may be helpful to indicate on the plan the approximate times each task is expected to occur. However, according to Benner's novice to expert (1982) theory, as novice learners students may attempt to strictly adhere to this organized routine. This inflexibility may hamper their success in acute placement settings where flexibility is essential. Therefore, when providing students with a skeleton schedule for clinical shifts, such as the one outlined, it might be best to provide minimal information or task-oriented items to enhance nursing student development. Note that the times provided here are only examples in an eight-hour clinical shift. CIs should adhere to a strict timeframe for pre- and post-clinical conferences and break times.

Figure 5.3 *Skeleton Schedule*

- 0650: Pre-conference and check in with CI
- 0700: Nursing handover from the previous shift (completed with your supervising nurse)
- 0715: Review orders, medication times, recent lab and test results, and upcoming procedures. Plan your nurse's brain (see the Clinical Learning Activity) and determine what your priorities are for the shift ahead.
- 0750: Room safety check
- 0800: Initial assessment, vital signs, and documentation
- 0900: Medications (completed with your CI or supervising nurse)
- 0945: Morning break (30 minutes)
- 1015: Nursing patient care, interventions, assessments; catch up on documentation, gather information for patient logs or assignments
- 1200: Lunch break (45 minutes)
- 1245: Ensure completion of any care, interventions, and documentation
- 1430: Handover to your supervising nurse
- 1500: Post-conference

Finally, CIs may find it helpful to stay a little later following the post-conference to wrap up any administrative work, check in with the staff nurses, and complete any evaluative tasks.

Clinical Learning Activity: Day Planners, Time Sheets, and a Nurse's Brain

CIs can provide nursing students with a day planner, also known as a time sheet or *nurse's brain*, as an organizational sheet to capture important patient information as they plan their clinical shift and prioritize care (Parkes, 2020). This activity also addresses some of the challenges that nursing students face in acute placement settings. The nurse's brain can prevent students from feeling lost and be a tool to aid in collaborating with their nurse preceptor when assigning tasks for the shift, communicating with members of the interprofessional team, and delivering a thorough yet concise and structured nursing handover report (Parkes, 2020).

As students begin to care for higher acuity or multiple patients, being familiar with a planner can help reduce anxiety and time-related pressures by providing them with an organized plan. Students are encouraged to develop their own nurse's brain that meets their own learning need and aligns with the workflow of the placement setting (see Figure 5.4 for the key components of a nurse's brain). These tools can also be valuable as students collect information for patient logs, care plans, reflections, and course assignments.

CIs may also consider developing their own organizational tool as they begin to supervise a group of nursing students on acute placement units. A time sheet can allow CIs to schedule when students will perform skills, conduct assessments that require supervision, or be evaluated. These time sheets can also serve as a method of informal documentation for students' summative and formative evaluation measures by identifying student learning needs and documenting experiences.

The CI is responsible for ensuring that students are aware that these brain sheets do not replace checking the chart for updated orders, reviewing the medication administration record, or completing legal documentation. Brain sheets are simply an organizational tool to help the student to plan their shift. It is imperative that students discard confidential patient information (i.e., name, date of birth, health information number, other identifying information) in the approved confidential waste manner before leaving the unit.

Figure 5.4 *Key Components of the Nursing Brain Sheet*

- Patient demographics
- Allergies, code status, isolation precautions, and other alerts
- Reason for admission, diagnosis, past medical history
- Important team members, most responsible care provider
- Times of medications, tests, procedures
- Recent lab or test results
- Lines, tubes, wires (IV access, fluids, O_2 therapy, telemetry, Foley catheter, etc.)
- Diet orders or restrictions (NPO status, low sodium diet, etc.)
- Key components of the head-to-toe assessment, frequency, and trend of vital signs
- To-do list items or other notes

Source: Based in part on Parkes (2020).

Common Medications, Diagnoses, Skills, and Unit-Specific Procedures

CIs may choose to provide students with an overview of common medications, diagnosis, skills, and procedures before their arrival at the clinical setting as part of their orientation experience. Students in acute placement settings have reported that being prepared for their first clinical placement assisted them in coping by reducing stress and anxiety (Al Shahrani, 2015). The common medications, diagnoses, skills, and procedures list should be brief (i.e., no more than three to five items per category) so as to not overwhelm students. When providing this information ahead of time, CIs should be clear as to which medications on the list students can and cannot administer, as well as which skills students can and cannot perform (see Figure 5.2).

Methods to help students become familiar with medications, diagnoses, and skills as they bridge the theory-practice gap during their time on the clinical unit include a personalized pocket reference tool or a patient log and care plan. These two clinical learning activities are described in further detail next.

Clinical Learning Activity: Personalized Pocket Reference Tools

An activity that students have found helpful during their first acute clinical placement is keeping a notebook as a personalized reference tool. In this notebook, students record the meaning of terminology, details about medications, and information on diagnoses that come up during their placement (Al Shahrani, 2015). These pocket reference tools should be small enough to fit in a scrub pocket and will become a handy reference. CIs may choose to provide these notebooks and start to fill in information for students as a template. This approach demonstrates to students the type of information that is important to gather about a specific medication, diagnosis, skill, or term.

CIs can also direct students to the internet or social media sources, such as blog posts or video links, where nurses and students share different ways of creating a personalized pocket reference tool. For example, Nurse Liz (2019) shares her expertise on how to create a do-it-yourself reference notebook in a YouTube video.

CIs can have students create a personalized pocket reference tool as an engaging learning activity. CIs can provide colourful tabs, stickers, or pens for nursing students to use in making their guides. This activity could be part of the orientation process. While students are designing their guides, CIs can review the common medications used and diagnoses students should know before starting the practicum. Starting to create their pocket reference tools in a fun and safe classroom environment is an effective approach.

Many premade pocket and reference guides are available. Students may want to purchase one of these instead. These prefabricated and published pocket guides for student nurses often contain numerous tips to help with the stress of student clinical placements, in addition to information regarding the practical aspects of a clinical placement and information specific to various clinical settings (McGurk, 2018).

On the other hand, sometimes these premade guides are too bulky and cover a wide array of topics and acute practice areas. However, these guides may be a useful reference when students are creating their own concise pocket-sized reference tool. Using a premade tool to inform a personalized tool allows students to meaningfully bridge the theory-practice gap specific to their acute care practice experience. These tools can also be brought forward in future clinical placements and can serve as a journal for students to track their progress throughout their undergraduate nursing studies and new nursing careers.

Clinical Learning Activity: Patient Logs and Care Plans

Patient logs and care plans are used in both education and clinical practice to organize information about a patient's care and are tailored to meet the specific and unique needs of the patient, as well as identifying potential needs or risks (Vera, 2021). Fonteyn and Cahill (1998) and Sedlak (1992) are pioneering authors who demonstrated that the use of clinical logs and care plans by nursing students can identify learning needs and, in turn, improve students' clinical reasoning and judgement in practice. The objectives of patient logs and care plans are to empower students to actively engage in evidence-based nursing care that embodies a holistic approach to patient care while serving as a guide that harmonizes the patient's goals and role of the nurse (Vera, 2021).

For this reason, patient logs and care plans have long been used as a learning activity and assessment tool in baccalaureate education for nursing students, especially in the acute care placement setting (Fonteyn & Cahill, 1998; Sedlak, 1992). Patient logs and care plans are used to measure students' clinical judgement as students must demonstrate their ability to systematically "gather patient data, make sense of that data, provide appropriate care based on that data, and then evaluate both the patient's and one's own actions" (Bussard, 2018, p. 107).

Patient logs often follow a structured assessment tool or theoretical reflective thinking framework. For example, Tanner's (2006) thinking like a nurse framework focuses on clinical judgement through a process of noticing, interpreting, responding, and reflecting. If CIs are not provided with a patient log or assessment tool, they can use this framework to help guide students' critical judgement by deciding on a course of action in response to assessment findings and reviewing the outcomes of that action (Tanner, 2006). This process can be used as a measure for students to reflect both in-action and on-action, discussed later in this chapter. Bussard (2018) found that the thinking like a nurse model can be useful for student evaluation in high-fidelity simulation environments.

CIs should encourage students to use these assignments as a clinical learning activity beyond the assigned grade or expected evaluative tool and as a personal method to enhance their knowledge and apply to future patient care. CIs must be familiar with the academic requirements but also promote the use of this assessment tool as a way for students to meaningfully connect what they learn in the classroom with their acute care clinical experiences.

An example of nursing students making a meaningful assessment and demonstrating critical judgement in an acute care placement through the development of a patient log occurs when they identify an unexpected assessment finding. An example of an encounter may occur when a student discovers a swollen limb distal to an infusing intravenous site. Using patient logs allows students to make inferences about the meaning of their clinical findings and guides their actions as they learn to manage interstitial peripheral intravenous infusions and identify risk for extravasation injury. Further, students can use these logs for self-growth and awareness of their individual learning needs (Sedlak, 1992). CIs can use the student's documented encounter (the patient log or care plan) to assess student progress towards clinical judgement and ultimately the ability to provide safe, skilful, quality patient care (Bussard, 2018).

Documentation

Students are accountable for ensuring accurate and timely documentation of their assessments and interventions in the acute placement setting. Documentation ensures there is clear communication between all members of the health care team, fulfils legal obligations to ensure patient safety, and can be used for data for research and quality improvement initiatives (Goodwin, 2019). Whether the clinical practice setting uses electronic or paper charting systems, students are expected to document clear, comprehensive, objective, and accurate findings on the patient record in a timely fashion, in accordance with hospital, academic, and governing body guidelines (College of Nurses of Ontario [CNO], 2019; Goodwin, 2019). For an example of documentation guidelines, CIs can direct students to the CNO's *Practice standard: Documentation* (2019) four-part module. Clinical placement facilities may also have online learning modules for nursing student documentation as part of the orientation to charting systems.

Documentation completed by students is not unlike charting completed by staff nurses on the unit. Documentation should include assessment data, changes in patient condition, interventions, treatments provided, patient responses to treatments, and communication with family and health care team members (Goodwin, 2019). Each clinical setting dictates the minimum frequency with which students and staff nurses are expected to document patient assessment, vital signs, and complete nursing notes (Goodwin, 2019). Some facilities may use a flow-sheet-based charting system, whereas others use narrative nursing notes, or a combination of both. Many health care facilities have now transitioned to electronic charting systems, and these can vary between regions. It is up to the CI to be familiar with the charting expectations and guidelines and to monitor student documentation in the facility-specific format.

Written errors and forgotten information are two of the simplest (yet most common) aspects of documentation that CIs must address with students (Goodwin, 2019). Handwritten documentation must be in blue or black ink, and errors should be indicated with a single line drawn through them, followed by the initials of the documenting practitioner (Goodwin, 2019).

Students are also expected to sign their documentation, using a nursing student identification as per their academic institution guidelines. Often, in addition to their name, a student signature indicates their designation as a nursing student, the name of their academic institution, and their level of experience. For example: *J. Doe, Level 3 nursing student, ABC University*

Some documentation and charting may require co-signature by an RN. This RN may be the supervising staff nurse or the CI. CIs need to be aware of any unit-specific requirements for this co-signing and communicate these mandatory documenting expectations to the students and supervising staff RN. Electronic systems should indicate the nursing student profile as an automated process. It is up to the CI to verify that signing and any co-signing have occurred.

To ensure that patients receive timely and efficient care, CIs can compare students' assessment documentation with charting done by an RN on the unit. This comparison, when it involves the student and an RN collaborating, can illustrate the importance of identifying changes in a patients' condition, documenting that change promptly, and completing tasks in a timely manner (Ironside et al., 2014). Encouraging students to carefully review charting done by staff nurses may also serve as a reminder of additional tasks that still need to be done.

Beyond the Checklist

Traditional task completion, in alignment with Benner's (1982) novice to expert theory, can often be a main focus of learning in acute placement settings (Ironside et al., 2014). Ironside et al. (2014) found that students were aware of the centrality of task completion and therefore often declined other learning experiences because they were concerned these may interfere with the timeliness of their patient care, rather than viewing additional opportunities as a chance to enhance their learning. CIs need to advocate for students' learning and ensure that these additional learning opportunities are not missed. CIs may need to give students permission to step away from the day-to-day patient care tasks to participate in unique learning opportunities that will enhance their experience in the acute placement setting.

Students found that focusing on fundamental tasks and activities of daily living (such as ensuring completion of hygiene care) could distract them from participating in additional learning opportunities (Annear et al., 2014). CIs need to facilitate student learning beyond the checklist by frequently checking in with students and supervising nurses to ensure that students are practising to their full scope and seeking additional learning experiences. For example, students may find observing procedures that are beyond their scope to be rich learning experiences that should not be missed (Ironside et al., 2014).

Bristol (2021) suggests that medication administration is not the most important aspect of the clinical experience and that focusing on this technical skill could take away time for students to engage in clinical reasoning activities. They suggest CIs have students administer only two or three medications during a clinical shift to allow time to focus on deeper learning and critical thinking activities (Bristol, 2021). Should the clinical facility or academic institution permit, students could also participate in medication administration under direct supervision from the precepting staff nurse (rather than the CI). The medication administration experience should include a focus on critical reasoning skills that accompany this task.

Another example of moving beyond the checklist occurs when a patient requires venipuncture for blood work. The CI can engage the student in helping the supervising nurse gather the supplies and in learning the order of blood collection. Although students are not to perform the venipuncture themselves, students become actively involved in the learning process when they are invited to participate in various aspects of a task-based competency that is out of their scope of practice. Beyond the checklist, students can observe the supervising nurse or phlebotomist's technique, follow up with the results of the blood test, and participate in a discussion that includes a critically reasoned interpretation of results and anticipated nursing actions.

Filling in Down Time

Occasionally, students may find themselves with spare time after completing all their assigned patient tasks, including assessments, medications, interventions, and documentation. Students should be encouraged to check in with their assigned RN or with the CI to seek out additional learning opportunities on the unit. Skills review and practice are especially useful, and rehearsals of an anticipated skill can help boost confidence and allow students to prepare for success in the clinical setting (Lundberg, 2008). Even helping classmates, or their preceptor, with activities of daily living with their patients shows initiative and should be encouraged.

Should students exhaust all possible patient care activities, CIs can have students fill this down time with information gathering for patient logs, care plans, or assignments. However, CIs should caution nursing students not to use this time to complete assignments if it is an academic expectation that the assignment be completed as homework. Students must embrace any learning opportunity that is unique to the placement setting and cannot be done elsewhere. Examples of learning opportunities that must be completed on site include completing learning modules that are only accessible on the hospital's internal website or computer system, attending in-service education sessions such as mock codes, or attending in-service briefings on a new piece of technology.

When a student often experiences down time, this should indicate to the CI that the student is ready for a heavier patient assignment. This could include taking on an additional patient or caring for a more complex or acute patient. See the Developing Patient Assignments section earlier in this chapter for further details.

Supporting the Preceptor

As previously discussed, a key CI role is to facilitate a welcoming relationship between the students and supervising staff nurses. The supervising staff nurse is sometimes termed the preceptor. Beyond their work with students, CIs should also provide support to preceptors to help maintain a healthy relationship in which they feel valued and respected for their extra effort and for the support they provide students (Courtney-Pratt et al., 2011).

In acute care placement settings, the nursing student experience is influenced by multiple factors, such as their relationships with their preceptors (Courtney-Pratt et al., 2011). Courtney-Pratt et al. (2011) found that preceptors are often initially reluctant to take on the role because of lack of confidence resulting from limited experience, heavy workloads, and time constraints. The business of acute placement settings can limit a preceptor's ability to spend time teaching students (Courtney-Pratt et al., 2015).

CIs should regularly check in with preceptors and with students to informally evaluate their comfort with their relationship and with the quality of their learning experience. Preceptors have reported that when they are given positive feedback, they are eager to participate as a preceptor again. This feedback reinforces how much knowledge they must share (Courtney-Pratt et al., 2011). When preceptors are effectively supported by CIs, a positive learning opportunity for both preceptors and students occur. A positive relationship between the academic institution and the placement setting is helpful to future students.

Expect the Unexpected: Uncertainties in Acute Care Settings

Acute care practice settings offer unique learning opportunities for students. Students can apply their theoretical classroom learnings to real-time patient care. Currently, patient acuity is increasing as patients have more comorbidities and are living longer with advancements in technology. Therefore, CIs need to be prepared and equipped to help students navigate these expected unexpected situations, helping to frame them as motivating learning experiences for future practice. Students are not expected to solely, and proficiently, manage unexpected occurrences in the acute care placement setting. Rather, students should be prepared to ask for help and to feel comfortable doing so. CIs should anticipate possible unexpected occurrences that students may confront and prepare students for these. Skills with observation, communication, conflict resolution, reflection, and handling errors are important to develop in advance of unexpected events.

Patient Deterioration, High Acuity, Code Blue

Students are expected to keep their preceptor and the CI regularly updated on their patient's status, planned interventions, and medications administered (Akuamoah-Boateng, n.d.). CIs must regularly check on patients for whom students provide care. CIs should introduce themselves to the patient and their family as the supervising CI. Students are obligated to inform their patients of their nursing student status and the name of their supervising staff nurse and CI so patients feel confident receiving care from a pre-service learner. It is imperative that CIs foster a supportive environment that facilitates students' reporting any changes in a patient's condition so that subtle signs of patient decompensation do not go unnoticed.

If a nursing student is caring for a patient whose clinical status deteriorates throughout the course of the shift, the precepting nurse is expected to take over the care of the patient (Akuamoah-Boateng, n.d.). Remember, students are supernumerary. If there is patient deterioration, students can be invited to observe the ongoing care and to participate as delegated by their supervising nurse if the assigned task is within their scope (i.e., priming IV fluids, documenting vital signs). The CI should be present if the student is assisting in these high-acuity moments to lend practical task-based support and emotional support to the student. Alternatively, a student can be reassigned to other patients (Akuamoah-Boateng, n.d.); however, it is best if students stay involved in the care of a decompensating patient as this can be an important learning experience unique to practice-based learning in acute care practicums

Communication Is Key

Clear, concise communication reduces errors, promotes team functioning, and improves interpersonal morale in acute placement settings. Clear, concise communication using acronyms or communication tools, especially in unexpected situations, ensures that consistent messaging is conveyed. For example, routine use of the SBAR technique (see the Clinical Learning Activity: SBAR, below) reinforces students' development of professional communication skills (Thomas et al., 2009). CIs should engage students regularly in SBAR-style communication, even in routine communication encounters, so that students are prepared to confidently and concisely communicate any concerns during unexpected encounters.

CIs can further reinforce clear communication using SBAR by having students play the role of members of the health care team in scenarios. During these role-play activities, students communicate encounters from their clinical shift or from case studies. CIs who encourage nursing students to use SBAR during routine and acute scenarios teach nursing students to be key players of patient safety as they transition from academia to clinical practice (Thomas et al., 2009).

Clinical Learning Activity: SBAR

SBAR is an acronym that stands for situation, background, assessment, and recommendation. It is a communication technique developed to increase the quality and conciseness of communication, particularly during handoffs between providers (Institute for Healthcare Improvement, n.d.; Muller et al., 2018; Stewart & Hand, 2017). For acute placement settings, this tool can be applied to nurse-to-nurse handover, nurse-to-physician communication when describing a change in patient condition, and so forth. The objective of using SBAR is to increase patient safety by empowering providers at any level of care to communicate their concerns concisely and clearly. This type of communication is essential because communication breakdown is one of the leading causes of adverse events in acute clinical settings (Muller et al., 2018; Stewart & Hand, 2017).

The SBAR tool is available for download from the Institute for Healthcare Improvement (n.d.) and has been adapted for use by students in acute placement settings in Figure 5.5. In a simulated environment, students who were educated to communicate and collaborate using the SBAR technique reported an improvement in their ability to focus on patient safety when communicating with their peers (Fay-Hillier et al., 2012). The example below demonstrates how students may communicate a concern from their assessment to either their preceptor or to a physician.

Figure 5.5 *Adapted SBAR Tool*

SBAR category		Description	Example for nursing students in acute placement settings
S	Situation	A brief overview of the problem	"I am concerned that Mr. X may be displaying signs of a post-operative surgical infection."
B	Background	Pertinent and relevant contextual information related to the problem	"Mr. X was admitted to the ward yesterday on post-operative day 1 following an appendectomy."
A	Assessment	Considerations include an overview of the contributing factors of what you found or think is contributing to the problem	"Mr. X is febrile, tachycardic, has a delayed capillary refill time but is normotensive at this time. He remains alert and oriented x3 but complains of pain at his surgical incision site that does not improve with PRN analgesia medication. The surgical site is covered with a dressing with new purulent drainage present."
R	Recommendation	Conclusion, explicitly stating what you are requesting from the person in the collaboration	"Can you please come assess Mr. X and we can discuss any further interventions that may be required upon your arrival."

Source: Adapted from the Institute for Healthcare Improvement (n.d.).

Handling Errors

Errors in clinical practice are not uncommon among nursing students; however, the shock and associated feelings when students discover an error can be unexpected, especially in acute practice settings. In a clinical context, errors are defined as a mistake, an inadvertent occurrence, or an unintended event in the delivery of care which may or may not result in patient injury, harm, or death (Benner et al., 2002). A study by Henneman et al. (2010) found that in a simulated environment, 100% of nursing students committed medical errors. CIs and students have an obligation to the clinical facilities, academic institutions, regulatory bodies, and patients to report any errors. This reporting provides opportunity for learning and facilitates the necessary follow-up to ensure accountability is enforced, which is essential to maintaining public trust in health care systems (CNA, 2015).

Most errors in the acute placement setting occur as medication errors during administration (Asensi-Vicente et al., 2018). CIs must be equipped to handle the errors in a manner that supports the student's learning and emotional needs. As students develop experience and competencies in medication administration, a clear understanding of how to prevent, identify, and report errors in the clinical setting should be a key component of undergraduate nursing programs (Freeman et al., 2020). However, a qualitative study by Noland (2014) found that 50% of nursing student respondents were inconsistently trained on how to navigate handling medication errors, even though 100% were told they had to report their mistakes.

CIs foster the creation of a culture of safety for students. CIs should teach students about the types of mistakes that can occur, the expectations about how students report mistakes, and what students can expect from the follow-up when a mistake is reported. It has been well documented that students, especially in clinical settings, learn best when relating to others (Benner et al., 2002; Lin et al., 2014). Therefore, a useful teaching strategy is for CIs to relate to students by sharing details about errors they have made in the past, including details about how they felt and the processes they went through (Seyedrasooli et al., 2019). This sharing of experiences by the CI is not to diminish the seriousness of making an error; rather, it is an opportunity for growth through social learning and normalizes the unexpected experience and emotional accompaniment of making an error.

Nursing students are at risk of becoming secondary victims to medical errors in the clinical setting, particularly if they feel they are personally responsible and are traumatized by the event (Noland, 2014). When students are involved in a medical error, they often experience a range of emotions, most of which are negative. For example, panic, distress, fear, shame, guilt, anxiety, and fear of reporting the mistake to their CI (even though they value the learning experience) are common (Asensi-Vicente et al., 2018; Noland, 2014). CIs need to ensure that they provide emotional support to students to prevent secondary victimization when an error occurs. Providing a safe space can help students feel they are emotionally supported as they go through the reporting and follow-up processes. The expression of empathy will in turn allow students to learn from the experience and increases the likelihood that they will report any future errors or near misses.

Lin et al. (2014) shared a raw narrative written by a nursing student who recalls their experience with a medication error during an acute pediatric clinical placement. The student described the outcome as an overall positive learning experience as the CI was empathetic and understanding in trying to find out what happened using open, collaborative, and relatable conversation instead of assigning blame (Lin et al., 2014).

Students also need to have a clear understanding that errors are rarely caused by a single factor or individual and are often a result of a combination of system and human factors (Benner et al., 2002; Noland, 2014). Linking the reporting of an error to being professional, accountable, and responsible helps the student and others learn from the experience and can lead to changes in practice to prevent similar errors in the future (Benner et al., 2002).

Finally, given the likelihood that students will make mistakes in acute placement areas, new CIs also need to be prepared for mistakes (Seyedrasooli et al., 2019). Dealing with a student mistake is as stressful for the CI as it is for the student; however, mistakes are possible even in the presence of the best educators (Seyedrasooli et al., 2019). Using problem-based focused coping, CIs can take constructive steps to help change the situation, respond to the mistake in a calm and empathetic fashion, and focus on the positive growth and learning that occurs as a result (Seyedrasooli et al., 2019).

Conflict

Preceptorship and clinical placements in which students work alongside professionals may generate conflict, which is often due to communication and interpersonal problems (Mamchur & Myrick, 2003). If conflict is not challenged and resolved, negative outcomes can occur for students, CIs, and preceptors (Mamchur & Myrick, 2003). However, conflict does have the potential to stimulate personal growth for students, preceptors, and CIs, if it is resolved in a constructive manner and considers perspectives from all parties involved (Mamchur & Myrick, 2003). It is unrealistic for CIs to assume that conflict will not be present in an acute placement setting. Stress levels can be high as caregivers from diverse backgrounds come together to care for acutely ill patients. Members of clinical teams all bring different values, beliefs, and perspectives to the clinical environment. Therefore, to ensure that any encountered conflict does not detract from the students' experience, CIs need to ensure successful resolution is reached.

Conflict often arises from behaviours or attitudes that are perceived or experienced as disrespectful or disruptive (Altmiller, 2012). When students struggle to apply new and seemingly overwhelming information, they can experience *internal conflict*. Internal conflict occurs when a student experiences opposing values or beliefs within themselves that hampers their development as a person and as a nursing professional (MasterClass, 2020). By addressing the concerns, fears, and anxieties students experience and encouraging reflective thinking and the use of patient logs, CIs can help students navigate any internal conflict that may emerge.

Conflict that occurs between two individuals is described as *external conflict* and can be broken down based on the root of the cause of the conflict (MasterClass, 2020; Shonk, 2020). Task-, relationship-, and values-based conflict are sources of tension in the acute placement setting and can occur between two students, between a student and the CI, or between a student and the preceptor. In a study by Mamchur and Myrick (2003), 51% of students reported experiencing conflict between themselves and their preceptor "frequently" or "almost always." Chapter 2 discussed some of the conflict that members of student groups may experience during the storming stage of Tuckman's group process theory.

CIs act as mediators when students need to resolve conflict with others. They should make an intentional effort to identify and resolve the cause of any conflict as unresolved tensions can cause students to disconnect from the learning process (Altmiller, 2012). One source of conflict that students have reported is not having their questions answered (Altmiller, 2012). On the other hand, CIs or preceptors have, at times, become defensive when they perceived student questioning as a challenge to their practice (Altmiller, 2012). Practical efforts that CIs can make to navigate this situation are to be sensitive to any occurrence of what a party may perceive as conflict, to act immediately if they sense conflict, and to assume a proactive role in the conflict resolution process by valuing all perspectives in an action plan that focuses on the source of the conflict (Mamchur & Myrick, 2003).

Reflection-in-Action

Reflective thinking is a skill students learn to use to address concerns and to bridge the theory-practice gap (Peden-McAlpine et al., 2005; Suwanbamrung, 2015). Reflection-in-action is the first level of Schon's (1983) on-action theory, whereby learners and clinical practitioners intentionally reflect *during* a clinical situation or unexpected experience. Based on Dewey's (1933) progressive perspectives of adult education, reflection-in-action provides a framework for CIs and students to use intuitive technical problem-solving skills in real-time clinical environments (Peden-McAlpine et al., 2015; Sellars, 2017).

By actively reflecting in the moment, students can develop their ability to think critically and to perform effectively in acute placement settings. Nursing education leader Patricia Benner (1982) also recognized the importance of reflective thinking practices as a means to support students in acute care settings as they transition through the levels of proficiency. Benner (1982) theorized that novice nurses, including pre-service learners, are unable to use discretionary judgement and can minimally interpret the context of a situation because it is too new to them, causing them to focus on task performance.

CIs are responsible for facilitating the development of meaningful and practical knowledge, skill performance, and judgement in students through methodological and experience-based education as they progress through Benner's proficiency stages. Engaging students through in-action reflection is a pragmatic time- and cost-efficient teaching competency (Gordon, 2016). When unexpected encounters occur in the acute placement setting, students need to be able to adapt and implement critical thinking skills to safely address these concerns. Reflection-in-action facilitates the development of learner reflexivity which means students can begin to think ahead, analyze their experiences in the moment, and respond effectively to a given situation (Gordon, 2016).

One key component of learner reflexivity is the enhanced consciousness approach to clinical decision-making and reasoning (Afolayan, 2016). In the next section, the second part of Schon's (1983) on-action theory (reflection-on-action) is discussed.

Wrapping Up

Reflection-on-Action

Reflection-on-action is the *retrospective* practice of analyzing performance after an event to gain meaningful and tacit knowledge to apply to future practice (Rolfe, 2002; Schon, 1983). Concepts of behaviourism, constructivism, transformative learning, and social learning all contribute to the development of skill with reflection-on-action as a form of reflexive learning.

There are a multitude of on-action reflection frameworks that CIs can use to facilitate learner reflexivity following clinical encounters in the acute placement setting. For example, Rolfe (2002) built on the reflection-on-action framework using the critical reflective prompts of *what?*, *so what?*, and *now what?* Although a simple reflective framework, Rolfe's (2002) on-action reflective guide can be used by CIs to facilitate comprehensive application of thinking through situations and can be applied in a variety of formats, such as post-conference discussions, Socratic questioning during the debriefing process, or a formal written reflective journal. See Clinical Learning Activity: Reflective Journaling later in the chapter (Gordon, 2016).

CIs should encourage the use of a variety of different on-action reflective frameworks and mediums for communicating these on-action reflections. Students may find one method of reflection is best suited to their learning needs or to the context of the clinical encounter they are reflecting on. For example, one student may prefer to verbally reflect-on-action, whereas another in the same clinical group may prefer some form of artistic expression such as poetry to express reflection. Using a variety of reflection approaches gives CIs the opportunity to assess learners' level of comprehension and knowledge acquisition.

Post-Conference

Post-conference is a dedicated time immediately following a clinical shift when students and CIs collectively debrief and reflect-on-action their recent experiences. Successful post-conferences, much like pre-conferences, are built on the principles of invitational and transformative learning theory. CIs facilitate a protected environment where students can engage and consolidate their learning by making connections from theory to their recent clinical experiences. Post-conference is also an opportunity for students to share their experiences by way of storytelling, explore their feelings, and help them understand the patient-nurse relational experience (Hsu, 2007). CIs can use the structured and dedicated time of post-conference to assess students' comprehension and knowledge acquisition and to provide timely feedback to facilitate students' progress in meeting the course objectives.

The structure of successful post-conferences may vary based on the stage the clinical group is in (see Tuckman's group process theory in Chapter 2). CIs may want to begin organizing their clinical post conferences to include an opening with an icebreaker or light-hearted activity to bring students together as a group, followed by the sharing of stories or a debriefing session related to the recent clinical shift. Post-conferences could also include a key teaching point or interactive educational activity. Each clinical conference should conclude with a summary and identification of implications and learnings from the discussion that can be applied in upcoming clinical situations

(Gaberson et al., 2015). Extension of the clinical post-conference may need to occur, with one-on-one follow-up that supplements the small group discussion to resolve conflicts or address areas of concerns identified during the post-conference.

One recognized downfall of post-conferences is that students are often tired and exhausted after a clinical shift, when post-conferences are usually held (Bristol, 2021; Yehle & Royal, 2010). When students are required to sit in a small room and engage in in-depth conversations and active listening, it can contribute to clinical fatigue (Bristol, 2021). To minimize this fatigue, clinical post-conferences should be part of the time students are scheduled to be at the clinical facility and held in a private area to help maintain student motivation and energy. Including active learning activities in the post-conference may help students stay engaged and alert (Yehle & Royal, 2010). Some suggested clinical activities for post-conference (including components of debriefing and meaningful storytelling) are described in further detail next (see also Figure 5.6).

Figure 5.6 *Clinical Learning Activities for Post-Conference*

- ***Nursing handover:*** Pair up students and have them give each other a report as if they were handing off to the next shift (Bristol, 2021).
- ***Minute to win it:*** Divide students into groups to practise acute clinical skills that may have been part of the recent shift or that you anticipate occurring during an upcoming shift (Yehle & Royal, 2010). These activities take no more than two minutes to complete and should encourage healthy competition. Examples include medication calculations, IV fluid priming, or a matching game (e.g., medication to drug class or clinical indication), and so on.
- ***Practice NCLEX questions:*** Prepare 5 to 10 NCLEX-style questions that apply to the placement setting (Yehle & Royal, 2010). Review the questions with your students and discuss the answers and rationale using experiences from the acute placement setting, as well as theoretical knowledge.
- ***Journal club:*** Have one or two students each week find a recent journal article that applies to the acute placement setting. This activity encourages students to practise evidence-based care in real-time clinical placement settings.
- ***Interprofessional presentations:*** Invite a member of the interprofessional team to come to give a short presentation about their role in the placement setting. This activity will also acquaint students with various team members and help them feel welcomed into the unit culture.

Debriefing

Debriefing is a common practice in pre-service nursing education, particularly in simulation settings. Debriefing also occurs in real-time clinical practice, often after a critical event and with various members of the interprofessional team (Toews et al., 2021). However, debriefing also serves as a meaningful tool for pre-service learners as a routine component of a post-conference, particularly in acute placement settings where unexpected or acute situations occur. CIs should incorporate debriefing in their clinical education practice as a component of the post-conference discussion to openly facilitate a guided discussion and collective reflective practice among their group of students.

CIs need to have a purpose and goal before beginning a debriefing session. The purpose can be as simple as summarizing a clinical shift, addressing any areas of concern, resolving conflicts, discussing an unexpected event, or highlighting a key area of practice such as the trajectory of a patient diagnosis. Toews et al. (2021) described five attributes of a clinical debriefing session that CIs can use to help guide the session: experienced/educated facilitator, environment, education, evaluation, and emotions. *Equality* is a sixth E that should be added to this model. Equality means each student and involved party should have equal opportunity to contribute to the debriefing conversation so that all students can be active participants and enjoy the benefits of clinical debriefing. As skilful facilitators, CIs can redirect and engage all students in conversation by encouraging them to share their experiences or perspectives to examine different points of view and arrive at solutions (Gaberson et al., 2015). Having a purposeful debriefing session allows the CI to ensure that the dialogue is focused, sidetracks are avoided, and time is managed (Gaberson et al., 2015). However, the planned debriefing structure should not deter from organic conversations that stimulate the development of students' clinical reasoning or reflective practices.

When debriefing activities feel psychologically safe, they can help students validate their ideas and ways of processing information. As students learn to express emotions openly, they begin to develop reflective practice, higher-level thinking, clinical reasoning, and judgement skills (Toews et al., 2021). Socratic questioning, in which the CI does not answer students' questions directly but uses tenets of inquiry to stimulate critical reflection and problem solving, can also strengthen debriefing activities (Dreifuerest, 2015; Gaberson et al., 2015). Questions to facilitate debriefing can be guided by a reflective framework such as Rolfe's (2002) on-action reflective framework, which uses the prompts of *what?*, *so what?*, and *now what?* Other facilitative questions include identifying the *who*, *what*, *when*, *where*, *why*, and *how* of a clinical situation (Dreifuerest, 2015). A prompt that CIs can use during debriefing discussion is "Tell me more." This prompt is effective when conversation stops or to draw out a quieter nursing student.

Regardless of the approach used to structure a purposeful debriefing process, the final evaluative component of the session must conclude by summarizing what was learned and noting the implications for future practice (Dreifuerest, 2015). During the evaluation phase of the debrief, students actively demonstrate learner reflexivity, identify learning goals and opportunities for future patient care and clinical encounters, set attainable goals, and re-evaluate their practice (Dreifuerest, 2015; Toews et al., 2021). In the acute placement setting, students may be able to engage in higher order thinking as they anticipate future situations (Dreifuerest, 2015).

Finally, CIs can use the final component of the debriefing process to address and resolve any remaining conflicts. Students may have concerns that require follow-up in a more intimate meeting, rather than in a group setting (Toews et al., 2021).

Storytelling

Reflective thinking practices are not solitary; rather they involve sharing clinical experiences with others (Suwanbamrung, 2015). A cross-sectional survey by Dafogianni et al. (2015), shows that most students who experienced positive pediatric clinical placements were taught by instructors who encouraged open dialogue and empowered their self-confidence. Students found that this reflective, open communication resolved concerns they faced in the clinical environment (Dafogianni et al., 2015).

Students require frequent opportunities to share their experiences with their peers and with the CI in the form of unstructured storytelling (Lundberg, 2008). By relating their experiences in the acute clinical placement setting, students can develop realistic expectations regarding their progress with clinical skills, knowledge, and judgement within the context of social learning (Lundberg, 2008). In turn, hearing stories from experienced nurses in similar situations can ease students' feelings of isolation and contribute to their professional socialization.

Sharing raw, unstructured narratives that recount both positive and negative clinical stories is cathartic and can help students feel supported (Lin et al., 2015). Storytelling offers an opportunity for immediate feedback from peers, CIs, or experienced nurses. It can reinforce students' ability to function as a nurse and serve as a form of peer modelling in which fellow students can witness how their peers worked through difficult and unexpected situations (Lundberg, 2008). In post-conference settings, storytelling discussions can be gently guided away from perpetuating negative groupthink focused on failure and towards viewing experiences as optimistic learning opportunities.

Goal Setting

As previously mentioned, the final evaluative component of a debriefing session includes goal setting. This is an opportunity for students to set goals for future practice as they look ahead to reflection-beyond-action (Dreifuerst, 2015). Post-conference clinical discussions and activities provide students an opportunity to assess their own learning, identify gaps in their cognitive understanding, and learn from others in a non-evaluative environment (Gaberson et al., 2015). A common method of goal setting that students and CIs may be familiar with is the **SMART** method. Generating a meaningful objective that is **s**pecific, **m**easurable, **a**ttainable/achievable, **r**ealistic, and **t**imebound promotes the success and ongoing development of students in acute placement settings (Doran, 1981). CIs should review goals students develop for the short term (e.g., upcoming clinical shifts), mid-term (e.g., in time for a formative evaluation or end of the semester), and long term (e.g., for their clinical development as a future RN). Generating SMART goals will ensure that the course learning objectives of the acute placement setting are aligned with each student's individual objectives for their longer-term career goals. Collaborating with students to achieve their SMART goals makes the acute placement setting more personalized and enhances motivation to learn. Chapter 7 provides more details on how CIs can facilitate goal setting.

Evaluation

CIs should familiarize themselves with the evaluation tools and requirements from their academic facility before beginning a clinical practicum. CIs are responsible for assessing students' comprehension and knowledge acquisition in the clinical setting. Providing timely and effective feedback to students that facilitates their progress in meeting the course objectives is imperative. Effective feedback from CIs will also support the development of students' reflexive learning process as they are able to accept criticism and feedback and use it to produce tangible ideas for their future practice (Afolayan, 2016). There are two contexts for providing effective feedback and evaluative measures: summative and formative. CIs should be comfortable with and routinely perform both in the acute placement setting. For more information on these evaluative techniques, please refer to Chapter 7. Two clinical learning activities follow that CIs can implement as both formative and summative evaluation tools in acute placement settings. Ideally, these evaluation approaches can be used during the dedicated post-conference as part of the summary/conclusion phase of the debrief.

Clinical Learning Activity: Reflective Journaling

The reflective practice of journaling is the creation of a written document in which students analyze their thoughts, actions, or interactions in clinical practice by using guided reflection (Gonzalez-Garcia et al., 2020). Journals are also an effective reflective tool for students as they log their successes and monitor previous accomplishments (Lundberg, 2008). Journaling provides CIs with opportunities to offer positive feedback and comments that guide the development of realistic learning goals in these advanced settings (Lundberg, 2008; Mirlashari et al., 2017).

When students engage in self-reflection, they are empowered to voice emotions they experience during their placement related to their own individual context (Gonzalez-Garcia et al., 2020). Journaling encourages students, as pre-service learners, to recognize their own skill acquisition by incorporating evidence-based reflective practices. This process can be therapeutic for students and should therefore also be encouraged as a non-evaluative tool, allowing students to externalize their experiences to prepare them to face future difficulties or unexpected situations (Gonzalez-Garcia et al., 2020).

Clinical Learning Activity: Three Great Things

Three Great Things is a reflective practice activity that CIs can employ to provide structured and consistent feedback. The primary assumption of this activity is that the environment instructors create affects learning. This assumption draws on Gottman's (1994) balance theory, which was initially developed in the context of relational counselling to motivate people to continue doing what they were doing well. The activity also integrates the positive conditioning inherent in Bandura's (1977) social learning theory (Zenger & Folkman, 2013). CIs can invite nursing students to self-identify three positive actions they took and one opportunity for improvement. This pragmatic, cost-, and time-efficient approach provides students with ongoing positive feedback as they develop self-confidence, develop critical thinking skills, and ensure safe patient care in placement settings.

To provide effective feedback when using Three Great Things, CIs need to consistently use the 3:1 ratio of positive to constructive feedback as it has been demonstrated to be effective for behaviour change and goal setting for long-term learning (Gottman, 1994). By clearly and respectfully communicating performance expectations on a consistent basis, in a way that positive reinforcement outweighs criticisms, patient safety events are decreased, and learners are more receptive to feedback (Bedi, 2018).

When implementing Three Great Things in-action, CIs can prompt nursing students by saying, "As you perform this skill, consider three things that are going well and one aspect you want to learn more about or do differently." This approach invites students to practise optimistic reflective thinking while involved in acute clinical encounters. As previously discussed, reflection on-action occurs retrospectively and thus Three Great Things can be facilitated either immediately following a clinical encounter or unexpected event, during a post-conference to reflect on a clinical shift, or during summative one-to-one evaluation at the end of a semester. When using Three Great Things to facilitate reflective feedback, CIs cultivate a collaborative, reflective environment that fosters trust and reliability in the feedback process.

Summary

CIs are essential for the smooth integration of nursing students into acute care placement settings in preparation for entry to nursing. Successful integration of nursing students into these settings using a practice-based learning approach requires CIs to provide a thoughtful and thorough orientation process that welcomes students to a fast-paced clinical environment. Getting to know students allows CIs to liaise between the academic requirements and clinical placement expectations, and to manage student human factors over the term. In this chapter, the foundations of leading a group of nursing students in an acute care practicum were described. CIs were encouraged to develop the knowledge and skills to conduct pre- and post-conferences, develop patient assignments, fulfil legal documentation obligations, and organize a typical nursing shift on their assigned acute placement unit. CIs must also be equipped to handle the uncertainties and unexpected encounters that are inevitable in acute care practice settings. How CIs manage conflict resolution, facilitate in- and on-action reflective thinking practices, and support student experiences during a patient deterioration event or medical error are paramount to ensuring successful practice-based learning outcomes. Finally, CIs provide both formative evaluation and informal feedback to nursing students to shape their progression and skill development as the future generation of acute care nurses.

Conclusion

This chapter explored some of the unique challenges or unexpected occurrences that students may face in acute care placement settings. By having a strong understanding and foundational knowledge related to acute care clinical practicums, CIs can help nursing students use these challenges as learning opportunities that will shape their future practice. Clinical learning strategies and foundational skills were described that CIs can integrate into the clinical practicum learning, ensuring the development of learner reflexivity while safeguarding the delivery of patient care.

References

Afolayan, G. E. (2016). Reflexive learning. In S. L. Danver (Ed.), *The SAGE encyclopedia of online education*. Sage. https://doi.org/10.4135/9781483318332.n303

Akuamoah-Boateng, M. (n.d.). *Nursing clinical instructor: Quick guide*. Baycrest. https://www.baycrest.org/Baycrest/Education-Training/Students-Trainees/CI-Quick-Guide.aspx

Al Shahrani, Y. (2015). *Factors that assist undergraduate nursing students to cope with the experience of their first clinical placement* [Master's thesis, University of Adelaide]. Adelaide Research & Scholarship Repository. https://hdl.handle.net/2440/103030

Altmiller, G. (2012). Student perceptions of incivility in nursing education: Implications of educators. *Nursing Education Perspectives*, 33(1), 15–20. https://doi.org/10.5480/1536-5026-33.1.15

Annear, M., Lea, E., & Robinson, A. (2014). Are care workers appropriate mentors for nursing students in residential aged care? *BMC Nursing*, 13(1), 44. https://doi.org/10.1186/s12912-014-0044-8

Asensi-Vicente, J., Jimenez-Ruiz, I., & Vizcaya-Moreno, F. (2018). Medication errors involving nursing students: A systematic review. *Nurse Educator*, 43(5), E1–E5. https://doi.org/10.1097/nne.0000000000000481

Bandura, A. (1977). Self-efficacy: Toward a unifying theory of behavioural change. *Psychology Review*, 84(2), 241–249. https://doi.org/10.1037//0033-295x.84.2.191

Bedi, S. (2018). *5:1 feedback improves medical care*. Air Force Medical Service. https://www.airforcemedicine.af.mil/News/Display/Article/1499653/51-feeedback-improves-medical-care/

Benner, P. (1982). From novice to expert. *American Journal of Nursing*, 82(3), 402–407.

Benner, P., Sheets, V., Uris, P., Malloch, K., Schwed, K., & Jamison, D. (2002). Individual, practice, and system causes of errors in nursing: A taxonomy. *The Journal of Nursing Administration*, 32(10), 509–523. https://doi.org/10.1097/00005110-200210000-00006

Bristol, T. (2021). *Five things I wish I had known before teaching clinical*. Elsevier Education. Retrieved June 2021 from https://evolve.elsevier.com/education/expertise/active-learning/five-things-i-wish-i-had-known-before-teaching-clinical/

Bussard, M. (2018). Evaluation of clinical judgment in prelicensure nursing students. *Nurse Educator*, 2(43), 106–108. https://doi.org/10.1097/NNE.0000000000000432

Canadian Association of Schools of Nursing. (2012). *Ties that bind: The evolution of education for professional nursing in Canada from the 17th to the 21st century.*

Canadian Interprofessional Health Collaborative. (2010). *A national interprofessional competency framework*. http://ipcontherun.ca/wp-content/uploads/2014/06/National-Framework.pdf

Canadian Nurses Association. (2015). *Framework for the practice of registered nurses in Canada*. http://elections.cna-aiic.ca/-/media/cna/page-content/pdf-en/framework-for-the-pracice-of-registered-nurses-in-canada.pdf

CASN Clinical Instructor Nurse Educator Interest Group. (2015). *Strategies for instructor activities*. https://www.casn.ca/wp-content/uploads/2015/02/Clinical-interest-group-document-2015-FINAL.pdf

College of Nurses of Ontario. (2019). *Practice standard: Documentation, revised 2008*. https://www.cno.org/globalassets/docs/prac/41001_documentation.pdf

College of Registered Nurses of Manitoba. (2018). *Practice direction: Assignment and delegation to unregulated care providers*. https://www.crnm.mb.ca/uploads/document/document_file_40.pdf

Courtney-Pratt, H., FitzGerald, M., Ford, K., Marsden, K., & Marlow, A. (2011). Quality clinical placements for undergraduate nursing students: A cross-sectional survey of undergraduates and supervising nurses. *Journal of Advanced Nursing, 68*(6), 1380–1390. https://doi.org/10.1016/j.nedt.2015.11.013

Dafogianni, C., Alikari, V., Galanis, P., Gerali, M., & Margari, N. (2015). Nursing student's views on their clinical placement in pediatric hospitals of Athens, Greece. *International Journal of Caring Sciences, 8*(3), 673–682. https://doi.org/10.1016/j.nedt.2013.02.007

Dewey, J. (1933). *How we think: A restatement of the relation of reflective thinking to the educative process.* Health & Company.

Doran, G. T. (1981). There's a S.M.A.R.T. way to write management's goals and objectives. *Management Review, 70* (11), 35–36. https://community.mis.temple.edu/mis0855002fall2015/files/2015/10/S.M.A.R.T-Way-Management-Review.pdf

Dreifuerest, K. T. (2015). Getting started with debriefing for meaningful learning. *Clinical Simulation in Nursing, 11,* 268–275. https://doi.org/10.1016/j.ecns.2015.01.005

Fay-Hillier, T. M., Regan, R. V., & Gallagher, G. M. (2012). Communication and patient safety in simulation for mental health nursing education. *Issues in Mental Health Nursing, 33*(11), 718–726. https://doi.org/10.3109/01612840.2012.709585

Fonteyn, M. E., & Cahill, M. (1998). The use of clinical logs to improve nursing students' metacognition: A pilot study. *Journal of Advanced Nursing, 28*(1), 149–154. https://doi.org/10.1046/j.1365-2648.1998.00777.x

Freeman, M. A., Dennison, S., Giannotti, N., & Voutt-Goos, M. J. (2020). An evidence-based framework for reporting student nurse medication incidents: errors, near misses and discovered errors. *Quality Advancement in Nursing Education, 6*(3). https://doi.org/10.17483/2368-6669.1233

Gaberson, K.B., & Oerman, M. H. (1999). *Clinical teaching strategies in nursing.* Springer Publishing Company. https://doi.org/10.1891/9780826140036

Gaberson, K., Oermann, M., & Shellenbarger, R. (2015). Discussion and clinical conference. In *Clinical teaching strategies in nursing* (4th ed., pp. 231–252). Springer.

Gilbert, J., & Brown, L. (2015). The clinical environment – Do student nurses belong? A review of Australian literature. *Australian Journal of Advanced Nursing, 33*(1), 23–28. https://www.ajan.com.au/archive/Vol33/Issue1/3Gilbert.pdf

Gonzalez-Garcia, M., Lana, A., Zurron-Madera, P. Valcarcel-Alvarez, Y., & Fernandex-Feito, A. (2020). Nursing students' experiences of clinical practices in emergency and intensive care units. *International Journal of Environmental Research and Public Health, 17*(6), 5686. https://doi.org/10.3390/ijerph17165686

Goodwin, D. L. (2019). Documentation skills for nursing students. *Nursing Made Incredibly Easy! 17*(2), 16–21. https://doi.org/10.1097/01.NME.0000553096.31950.4b

Gordon, E. J. (2016). "The good, the bad and the ugly": A model for reflective teaching practices in coaching pedagogy. *Strategies, 30*(1). https://doi.org/10.1080/08924562/2016.1251866

Gottman, J. M. (1994). *What predicts divorce? The relationship between marital processes and marital outcomes.* Lawrence Erlbaum.

Health Alliance of MidAmerica LLC. (n.d.). Conducting pre- and post-conferences [Powerpoint presentation, PDF]. *Michigan Center for Nursing.* https://www.michigancenterfornursing.org/

Henneman, E. A., Roche, J. P., Fisher, D. L., Cunningham, H., Reilly, C. A., Nathanson, B. H., & Henneman, P. L. (2010). Error identification and recovery by student nurses using human patient simulation: Opportunity to improve patient safety. *Applied Nursing Research, 23,* 11–21. https://doi.org/10.1016/j.apnr.2008.02.004

Herdman, T. H. (2012). *Clinical nursing assignments: Are we teaching the most important skills?* NANDA International. https://nandainternational.typepad.com/nanda-international/2012/08/clinical-nursing-assignments-are-we-teaching-the-most-important-skills.html

Hsu, L. (2007). Conducting clinical post-conference in clinical teaching: A qualitative study. *Journal of Clinical Nursing, 16*(8), 1525–1533. https://doi.org/10.1111/j.1365-2702.2006.01751.x

Institute for Healthcare Improvement. (n.d.). SBAR tool: Situation-background-assessment-recommendation. http://www.ihi.org/resources/Pages/Tools/sbartoolkit.aspx

Ironside, P. M., McNeils, A. M., & Ebright, P. (2014). Clinical education in nursing: Rethinking learning in practice settings. *Nursing Outlook, 62*(3), 185–191. https://doi.org/10.1016/j.outlook.2013.12.004

Jamshidi, N., Molazem, Z., Sharif, F., Torabizadeh, C., & Kalyani, M. N. (2016). The challenges of nursing students in the clinical learning environment: A qualitative study. *The Scientific World Journal.* https://doi.org/10.1155/2016/1846178

Kozier, B., Erb, G., Berman, A., Snyder, S. J., Buck, M., Yiu, M., & Leeseberg Stamler, L. (2014). Nursing education in Canada. In *Fundamentals of Canadian nursing: Concepts, process, and practice* (3rd ed., pp. 27–39). Pearson.

Lin, F. Y., Wu, W. W., Lin, H. R., & Lee, T. Y. (2014). The learning experiences of student nurses in pediatric medication management: A qualitative study. *Nurse Education Today, 34,* 774–748. https://doi.org/10.1016/j.nedt.2013.08.004

Lundberg, K. M. (2008). Promoting self-confidence in clinical nursing students. *Nurse Educator, 33*(2), 86–89. https://doi.org/10.1097/01.NNE.0000299512.78270.d0

MacDonald, J., Paterson, K., & Waller, J. (2016). Nursing student's reflections on practice placement experiences. *Nursing Standard: Official newspaper of the Royal College of Nursing, 31*(10), 44–50. https://doi.org/10.7748/ns.2016.e10230

Mamchur, C., & Myrick, F. (2003). Preceptorship and interpersonal conflict: A multidisciplinary study. *Journal of Advanced Nursing, 43*(2). https://doi.org/10.1046/j.1365-2648.2003.02693.x

MasterClass. (2020). *What is conflict in literature? 6 different types of literary conflict and how to create conflict in writing.* MasterClass Articles. https://www.masterclass.com/articles/what-is-conflict-in-literature-6-different-types-of-literary-conflict-and-how-to-create-conflict-in-writing

Matheney, R. V. (1969). Pre- and post-conferences for students. *American Journal of Nursing, 69*(2), 2860269. https://doi.org/10.2307/3453961

McGurk, V. (2018). Clinical placements: Pocket guides for student nurses [Review]. *Nursing Standard, 32*(22). https://rcni.com/nursing-standard/opinion/reviews/clinical-placements-pocket-guides-student-nurses-125421

Melrose, S., Park, C., & Perry, B. (2015). The clinical learning environment. In *Creative clinical teaching in the health professions.* AU Press. https://clinicalteaching.pressbooks.com/chapter/chapter-three-the-clinical-learning-environment/

Mirlashari, J., Warnock, F., & Jahanbani, J. (2017). The experiences of undergraduate nursing students and self-reflective accounts of first clinical rotation in pediatric oncology. *Nurse Education in Practice, 25,* 22–28. https://doi.org/10.1016/j.nepr.2017.04.006

Montgomery, M. (2009). Student self-selection of clinical assignments. *Nurse Educator, 34*(2), 47–48. https://doi.org/10.1097/NNE.0b013e3181990d75

Morley, D., Alexander, A., Hewitt, J., Pearce, T., Suter, E., & Taylor, C. (2015). Student life – Hit the ground running. *Nursing Standard, 29*(22), 66. https://doi.org/10.7748/ns.29.22.66.s55

Muller, M., Jurgens, J., Redaelli, M., Klingberg, K., Hautz, W. E., & Stock S. (2018). Impact of the communication and patient hand-off tool SBAR on patient safety: A systematic review. *BMJ Open*, *8*(8), e022202. https://doi.org/10.1136/bmjopen-2018-022202

Murdoch, N. L., Epp, S., & Vinek, J. (2017). Teaching and learning activities to educate nursing students for interprofessional collaboration: A scoping review. *Journal of Interprofessional Care*, *31*(6), 744–753. https://doi.org/10.1080/13561820.2017.1346807

Nicholson, H. F. (1945). Education through clinical assignments: Suggestions for the head nurse interested in making the daily clinical assignment an important factor in advancing the students' knowledge and development. *The American Journal of Nursing*, *45*(12), 1055–1057. https://www.jstor.org/stable/3417022

Noland, C. (2014). Baccalaureate nursing students' accounts of medical mistakes occurring in the clinical setting: implications for curricula. *Journal of Nursing Education*, *53*(3), S34–S37. https://doi.org/10.3928/01484834-20140211-04

Nurse Liz. (2019, April 2). *DIY reference notebook for new nurses, nurse practitioners and students* [Video]. YouTube. https://www.youtube.com/watch?v=_Wcicn-OHSg

Parkes, C. (2020, June 22). *Nurse's brain, part 1: What is a nurse's brain?* Level Up RN. https://www.leveluprn.com/blogs/resources-for-nursing-students/nurses-brain-part-1

Peden-McAlpine, C., Tomlinson, P. S., Forneris, S. G., Genck, G., & Meiers, S. J. (2005). Evaluation of a reflective practice intervention to enhance family-centered care. *Journal of Advanced Nursing*, *49*(5), 494-501. https://doi.org/10.1111/j.1365-2648.2004.03322.x

Registered Nurses' Association of Ontario. (2016). *Practice education in nursing*. https://rnao.ca/sites/rnao-ca/files/SHWE_Practice_Education_BPG_WEB_0.pdf

Rolfe, G. (2002). Reflective practice: Where now? *Nurse Education in Practice*, *2*, 21–29. https://doi.org/10.1054/nepr.2002.0047

Schon, D. (1983). *The reflective practitioner: How professionals think in action*. Basic Books.

Sedlak, C. A. (1992). Use of clinical logs by beginning nursing students and faculty to identify learning needs. *Journal of Nursing Education*, *31*(1), 24–28. https://doi.org/10.3928/0148-4834-19920101-07

Sellars, M. (2017). Reflective practice. In *Reflective Practice for Teachers*. (pp. 1–24). https://uk.sagepub.com/sites/default/files/upm-binaries/59229_Sellars.pdf

Seyedrasooli, A., Zamanzadeh, V., Ghahramanian, A., & Tabrizi, F. (2019). Nursing Educators' Experiences Regarding Students' Mistakes in Clinical Settings. *Iran Journal of Nursing and Midwifery*, *24*(6), 462–468. https://doi.org/10.4103/ijnmr.IJNMR_46_19

Shonk, K. (2020, October 1). 3 types of conflict and how to address them. *PON Daily Blog*. https://www.pon.harvard.edu/daily/conflict-resolution/types-conflict

Smith, P. M., Spadoni, M. M., & Proper, V. M. (2013). National survey of clinical placement settings across Canada for nursing and other healthcare professions – Who's using what? *Nurse Education Today*, *33*, 1329–1336. https://doi.org/10.1016/j.nedt.2013.02.011

Spence Laschinger, H. K., Wong, C., Read, E., Cummings, G., Leiter, M., Macphee, M., Regan, S., Rheaume-Bruning, A., Ritchies, J., Burkoski, V., Grinspun, D., Gurnham, M. E., Huckstep, S., Jeffs, L., Macdonald-Rencz, S., Ruffolo, M., Shamian, J., Wolff, A., Young-Ritchie, C., & Wood, K. (2019). Predictors of new graduate nurses' health over the first 4 years of practice. *Nursing Open*, *6*(2), 245–259. https://doi.org/10.1002/nop2.231

Stewart, K. R., & Hand, K. A. (2017). SBAR, communication and patient safety: An integrated literature review. *MedSurg Nursing*, *26*(5), 297–305.

Suwanbamrung, C. (2015) Learning experience of student nurses through reflection on clinical practice: A case study in pediatric nursing, Southern Thailand. *Walailak Journal of Science & Technology, 12*(7), 623–629. http://wjst.wu.ac.th/index.php/wjst/article/view/1152

Tanner, C. A. (2006). Thinking like a nurse: A research-based model of clinical judgment in nursing. *Journal of Nursing Education, 45*(6), 204–211. https://doi.org/10.3928/01484834-20060601-04

Thomas, C. M., Bertram, E., & Johnson, D. (2009). The SBAR communication technique: Teaching nursing students professional communication skills. *Nurse Education, 34*(4), 176–180. https://doi.org/10.1097/NNE.0b013e3181aaba54

Toews, A. J., Martin, D. E., & Chernomas, W. M. (2021). Clinical debriefing: A concept analysis. *Journal of Clinical Nursing, 30*(11/12), 1491–1501. https://doi.org/10.1111/jocn.15636

University of Alberta. (2021). *Clinical placements*. Faculty of Nursing. https://www.ualberta.ca/nursing/programs/clinical-placements/index.html

University of British Columbia. (2016). *Scope of practice: Psychomotor skills for BSN students*. School of Nursing – Okanagan Campus. https://nursing.ok.ubc.ca/wp-content/uploads/sites/6/2016/02/BSN-Scope-of-Practice-Mar2017.pdf

van Iersel, M., Latour, C. H. M., van Rijn, M., deVos, R., Kirtschner, P. A., & Scholte op Reimer, W. J. (2020). How nursing students' placement preferences and perceptions of community care develop in a more 'community-oriented' curriculum: A longitudinal cohort study. *BMC Nursing 19,* 80. https://doi.org/10.1186/s12912-020-00473-3

Vera, M. (2021). *Nursing care plans (NCP): Ultimate guide and database*. Nurselabs. https://nurseslabs.com/nursing-care-plans/

Wink, D. (1995). The effective clinical conference. *Nursing Outlook, 43*(1), 29–32. https://doi.org/10.1016/s0029-6554(95)80041-7

Worrall, K. (2007). Orientation to student placements: Needs and benefits. *Pediatric Nursing, 19*(1), 31–33. https://doi.org/10.7748/paed2007.02.19.1.31.c4443

Yehle, K. S., & Royal, P. A. (2010). Changing the post clinical conference: New time, new place, new methods, equal success. *Nursing Education Perspectives, 31*(4), 256–258. https://pubmed.ncbi.nlm.nih.gov/20882870/

Zenger, J., & Folkman, J. (2013). The ideal praise-to-criticism ratio. *Harvard Business Review*. https://hbr.org/2013/03/the-ideal-praise-to-criticism.html

CHAPTER 6

Practice-Based Learning in Community Placements

Ruth Schofield & Genevieve Currie

This chapter provides teaching and learning strategies for clinical instructors who are supporting students in community placements. Integration of entry-level professional practice standards for community health nurses, entry-to-practice competencies for public health nursing, and principles of primary health care provide a foundational curriculum enabling clinical instructors to support student learning in community placements. This chapter recognizes community placements in both traditional and non-traditional settings, with greater emphasis on public health nursing.

Chapter Objectives

After completing the chapter, the reader will be able to
- describe the learning context for community health nursing clinical experiences
- define the unique clinical instructor roles in community health nursing
- summarize teaching and learning strategies for community health nursing education
- describe challenges and strategies encountered in clinical education in the community

Introduction

Clinical instructors (CIs) teaching community health nursing clinical courses strive to enable students to broaden their understanding of the registered nurse (RN) scope of practice and the role of the community health nurse (CHN). CHNs are distinctly positioned with a comprehensive understanding of health and factors that influence health, including the social determinants of health, primary health care, community-based care, and population health. Clinical community health nursing education provides opportunities for students to apply theoretical knowledge, practice standards, and models to practice situations to better understand the role and scope of CHNs. With a focus on health rather than illness, and the expansion from an individual perspective to include families, groups, communities, populations, and systems in multiple settings, the CI roles in this context are complex and unique. For example, CHN practice and competencies are less focused on manual skills and interventions for individual clients, and more focused on facilitating competency development to address population health outcomes, including

- supporting healthy public policy and principles of social justice
- using knowledge of population health, determinants of health, primary health care, and health promotion to achieve health equity
- using knowledge of health disparities and inequities to optimize health outcomes for all clients including Black people, Indigenous people, and migrant populations new to Canada
- applying strategies to optimize client health literacy

While CHNs work with individuals and families, the focus is always on improving population health outcomes to achieve health equity. This includes the application and integration of the knowledge, skills, and attitudes required for entry-level competencies, such as the following:

- knowledge (e.g., population health, health promotion, mental health, epidemiology, Indigenous ways of knowing)
- skills (e.g., assessment, data collection, analysis, evidence-based implementation, group facilitation skills)
- attitudes (e.g., integration of social justice approaches, commitment to health equity, Truth and Reconciliation Calls to Action, anti-racism, respect for diversity)

Community health nursing education prepares students for competency domains as community advocates, health public policymakers, health promotion and disease prevention practitioners, and community health researchers. These nursing roles are present in public health, home health care, primary health care, correctional care, parish nursing, outpost nursing, and outreach nursing, among others (Community Health Nurses of Canada [CHNC], 2019).

To fulfil these roles, a solid and current knowledge in community and public health nursing practice positions instructors to be effective educators. This chapter presents a background and history of community health nursing in undergraduate nursing education over multiple decades. The numerous learning contexts for practice, and specific roles for CIs supporting students in this clinical learning experience, are described. In addition, teaching and learning strategies necessary to support a quality learning experience are articulated. Last, challenges and strategies in community health clinical education are discussed.

Background and History of Community Health Nursing Clinical

Community health nursing is an umbrella term for various nursing practice areas, including public health, home health, primary care, and rural and remote community health nursing (CHNC, 2019). Specific aspects of the history of nursing education have impacted community health nursing education. As Chapter 1 identified, the origins of community health nursing education align with the beginning of nursing education in postsecondary institutions, such as universities, and with the 1918 influenza pandemic (Duncan et al., 2020). According to the recent account of 100 years of university education at the University of British Columbia, an academic nursing leader, Ethel Johns, in 1919 inspired the move of nursing education to universities (Duncan et al., 2020; Vukic & Dilworth, 2020). This was driven by Johns's vision that nurses needed the "breadth and depth [at the university level] to fulfil the social mandate of addressing people's health needs across the life span" (Duncan et al., 2020, p. 2). Hence the mandate of university nursing education supported the preparation of leaders in community health nursing through certificate programs, especially as public health nurses (PHNs) (Duncan et al., 2020; Vukic & Dilworth, 2020). Other universities, including Dalhousie University, McGill University, the University of Toronto, the University of Western Ontario, the University of Alberta, and the University of Montreal, also supported the addition of the bachelor of science in nursing (BSN) providing for university education in public health nursing (Tunis, 1996, pp. 120–122).

Nursing education in universities originally focused on public health nursing. The curriculum prepared educators and PHNs with knowledge in psychology, sociology, and sciences, followed by a focus on content specific to public health nursing (Duncan et al., 2020). Public health nursing content included health teaching, school health, prevention and control of communicable diseases, social work principles, and administrative and organizational principles (Duncan et al., 2020). Not surprisingly, differences between hospital-based and university-based nursing preparation contributed to tension among educators and nurses until integration was established in 1942 at the University of Toronto (Duncan et al., 2020). However, by 1960 a national study by Helen Mussallem found the standard of nursing education was inadequate in hospital-based preparation and recommended nurses be prepared at the same level of education as other health professionals with a baccalaureate degree (Duncan et al., 2020). With growing demands in the health care workforce and the health care system in both hospitals and community, and with increasing specialization over the next two decades, nursing leaders advocated for a baccalaureate degree as the entry-level registered nursing education (Duncan et al., 2020). By 1989, all provinces except Quebec adopted the BSN/BN as an entry-to-practice requirement. Hence, CI teaching of community health nursing clinical education continued in this context.

The requirement for baccalaureate preparation for PHNs was further emphasized by legislation in some Canadian jurisdictions. For example, the educational requirements for a PHN employee in Ontario health units is articulated in the *Health Protection and Promotion Act*. The act states that a person hired to be a PHN must be registered with a College of Nurses and have public health nursing education from a degree-granting institution. As a result of this legislation, the PHN title became protected for the RN classification. Pre-licensure baccalaureate nursing programs became accountable for including public health nursing in the curriculum.

Traditional and Non-traditional Settings

Traditional sites for public health nursing included public health nursing clinics, school health, home visitation programs, and programs focused on communicable diseases. The shift to baccalaureate preparation for RNs compounded the existing national and global shortage of traditional student placements in community settings

(Cohen & Gregory, 2009a; Pijl-Zieber & Kalischuk, 2011). An overview of community health nursing clinical education in Canada found that a shift was occurring from traditional community health placements, such as community health clinics and public health organizations, to non-traditional settings (Cohen & Gregory, 2009a). These non-traditional community settings included churches, schools, not-for-profit advocacy and service organizations, neighbourhood libraries, parent groups, shelters, and correctional institutions (Babenko-Mould et al., 2016; Cohen & Gregory, 2009a; Dietrich Leurer et al., 2011; Pijl-Zieber & Kalischuk, 2011; Pijl-Zieber et al., 2015; Williams et al., 2016). The focus of clinical learning in these non-traditional placement settings was community-oriented (socio-environmental perspectives, health promotion, and injury/illness prevention activities with population-level projects) versus community-based (acute, rehabilitative, and curative care in community settings) (Cohen & Gregory2009a; Phillips & Schofield, 2020). Therefore, the non-traditional settings provided unique opportunities for students to incorporate principles of social justice and health equity into their nursing practice. This community-oriented or neighbourhood-as-client focus in community health nursing clinical education continues today (Babenko-Mould et al., 2016; Phillips & Schofield, 2020) and is explored further under the section on learning context in this chapter.

Clinical Hours and Evaluation

Although anecdotal findings have been gathered, no recent formal community health nursing clinical education research on clinical hours used in BSN/BN programs in Canada exists. In 2009 Cohen and Gregory reported a range of 14 to 390 public health clinical hours (390 was over two courses), with an average of 146 hours for an academic term (Cohen & Gregory, 2009a). Anecdotal information continues to validate this range in clinical hours (Community Health Nurses of Canada [CHNC] Educators and Practitioners Network, 2019).

Methods for student evaluation are similar in acute care and community clinical placements and include learning plans/contracts, clinical performance evaluation, and written assignments, including reflections. A key difference in community health nursing clinical courses is that community assessment/planning/promotion projects are included and enable students to learn and apply the community health nursing process with a particular client population/aggregate in community settings (Babenko-Mould et al., 2016; Cohen & Gregory, 2009a; Pijl-Zieber et al., 2015).

Entry-to-Practice Competencies

Like the 1918 influenza pandemic, the SARS health crisis in 2003 propelled leaders in community health nursing education to strengthen undergraduate preparation in public health nursing. In 2012, CASN received funding from the Public Health Agency of Canada (PHAC) to develop *Entry-to-Practice Public Health Nursing Competencies for Undergraduate Nursing Education* (CASN, 2014). These competencies inform educational requirements for undergraduate students preparing for public health nursing practice. Similarly, the COVID-19 pandemic (beginning in 2020 and continuing into 2022) again highlights how essential it is to include community and public health nursing competencies in generalist nursing preparation and to provide all nursing students with the opportunity to develop entry-level competence in community and public health nursing.

In summary, for over a century, community and public health nursing clinical education has existed in the generalist baccalaureate preparation for RNs in Canada. The next section discusses unique aspects of the learning context and roles of CIs in community health nursing education placements.

Learning Context

The learning context in community health nursing education has characteristics not typically encountered within non-community-based courses. It is imperative that CIs are knowledgeable about these differences and grounded in community health nursing practice and standards of practice. The following areas should be considered by CIs when working with students in community health nursing education.

New Perspective of Client/Patient

CHNs work with clients that include individuals, families, communities, population groups, and larger systems. Community health nursing practice moves away from the reductionist and individualistic views of health that are centred on illness and disease models and individual responsibility. Instead, health is understood to be grounded in larger systems and structures and the relational interplay of political, economic, relational, and environmental forces that impact clients (Bekemeier & Butterfield, 2005; Kirkham & Browne, 2006). CIs have an important role in describing and recognizing the impact of these larger systems on health and in preparing students to critically analyze the relational, contextual, and intersectional impacts of systems on health for individuals, families, and communities (Falk-Rafael & Betker, 2012; Kirkham & Browne, 2006). For example, CIs can work with students to examine the impact of systems and health when working with individuals and community groups by analyzing population health data, examining the interplay of the social determinants of health, and interviewing community members to hear their perceptions of what factors impact their health (Quinn et al., 2019).

Non-structured or Minimally Structured Learning Environments

CIs must assist students to transition from structured acute care settings where there are many supports and resources in place, including others to hand off care to, to non-structured or minimally structured learning environments (Van Doren & Vander Werf, 2012; Williams et al., 2016). The non-structured or minimally structured learning environment can support students' proficiency in understanding and undertaking the entry-to-practice registered nursing competencies within the RN scope of practice. As discussed earlier, these community-oriented placement sites may include homeless shelters, schools and daycares, correctional centres, refugee centres, family support agencies, food banks, and worksites (Pijl-Zieber & Kalischuk, 2011). These sites can enrich students' understanding of the principles of primary health care (Canadian Nurses Association [CNA], 2015), allow them to see the impact of the social determinants of health (Lathrop, 2013; Reutter & Kushner, 2010), provide opportunities to work with diverse populations, and introduce the concepts of cultural humility (Fornoda et al., 2016) and cultural safety (Bourque Bearskin, 2011).

Students can acquire leadership skills in traditional and non-traditional community-based sites specific to health promotion orientation, systems thinking, collaborative working relationships, partnership building, and intersectoral collaboration (Bekemeier et al., 2015). Studies have found that it is important for students to work directly with individuals, families, and community representatives to gain a greater understanding of the structural/system barriers and facilitators experienced by individuals, which leads to increased empathy for equity-seeking groups (Ezhova et al., 2020). Being situated in non-structured or minimally structured learning environments can lead to role ambiguity and uncertainty for students, and this outcome will be discussed under challenges and strategies later in this chapter.

Community Health Practice Standards

According to a scoping review of community health nursing practice, inconsistencies exist in many nursing education programs in the use of models of practice and standards of practice (Ezhova et al., 2020). In Canada, community health nursing is grounded in the Canadian community health nursing [CCHN] professional practice model and standards of practice (CHNC, 2019) and the entry-to-practice public health nursing competencies for undergraduate nursing education (CASN, 2014), which are supported as national frameworks to guide curriculum development. These practice standards highlight the values, structure, and processes for providing care with clients within community settings and systems. CIs role-model and reinforce specific practice standards using the community health nursing professional practice model and standards of practice (CHNC, 2019). With the support of the practice model, CIs assist students to integrate these overarching standards and competencies into their nursing practice. These standards and competencies increase understanding of the expected practices and required knowledge, skills, and attitudes of nurses practising in the community and reduce role ambiguity within community health nursing.

Client-Centred and Strength-Based Approaches and Relational Practice

The mandate within community health nursing is working with clients (families, community partners, populations, and systems) where they reside and experience health and illness (Bekemeier et al., 2015). This moves away from focusing on illness management with individuals and expands to include population-based interventions and system change to improve health, reduce inequities, and increase access to health care. Embedded in this shift is building capacity for clients by using strength-based approaches (CHNC, 2019). A strength-based approach focuses on positives rather than deficits in knowing and working with the client. This approach also considers the whole person or community, what works well, and what resources exist to enable the client to deal more effectively with barriers to their health (Gottlieb, 2013). CHNs also embrace relational practice by providing care to clients as individuals, as well as families, communities, and populations, while adopting a larger view of the interplay with systems and health (CHNC, 2019). With a focus on providing nursing where clients live, work, and play, the nurse is more aware of factors that facilitate and impede health (Bekemeier et al., 2015). The nurse works with the client to reduce, eliminate, increase, or mitigate these factors. Thus, the CI must impart the importance of working with clients in their own space and place and using client-centred and strength-based approaches within interactions and interventions.

Sometimes, it can be unfamiliar and uncomfortable for students to move beyond an individualistic approach and consider upstream approaches to health (Falk-Rafael & Betker, 2012). As well, it can be difficult for students to let go of setting the daily schedule and determining the type and timing of interventions for clients, which often occurs in a hospital or acute care settings. CIs in community health nursing education recognize the importance of strong relationship-building skills when working with clients in determining priorities, sustaining contact to affect change, being culturally sensitive and respectful, and requesting input from clients into decisions and actions for promotion of health and prevention of illness/harm reduction (Ezhova et al., 2020). According to the scoping review by Ezhova et al. (2020), relationship-building skills are at the core of community health nursing practice and thus require development, reinforcement, and support from CIs.

Ethical Framework for Working with Individuals, Communities, and Populations

CIs draw students' attention to ethical frameworks used for decision-making in nursing within community settings. One such framework is the *Framework for Ethical Deliberation and Decision-Making in Public Health* developed by PHAC (2017). This framework addresses ethical issues in public health programs, policies, and other initiatives undertaken by public health providers. The framework provides a systematic approach using a five-step process in the analysis of challenges and dilemmas experienced while working in public health. Core ethical dimensions for public health include respect for persons and communities, non-maleficence and beneficence, trust, and justice. Procedural considerations include accountability, inclusiveness, responsibility, responsiveness, and transparency. Other ethical frameworks include the CNA Code of Ethics (2017), which provides national ethical standards for nursing. The National Collaborating Centre for Determinants of Health (NCCDH, 2020a, 2020b) also offers two ethical frameworks for students and providers to use when working with community members. These NCCDH frameworks specifically focus on health equity, including values and ethical foundations of health equity.

Health Inequities and Social Justice Actions

CIs are instrumental in guiding students to work in community-oriented settings where clients live, work, play, attend school, and age. Students have the unique opportunity to transition from institutionalized health care settings to witness social, political, economic, and environmental barriers experienced by clients in achieving equal health outcomes. In particular, students are more likely to encounter social and health disparities and inequities that are experienced by clients while working in settings where clients experience their daily lives. People experience social and health inequities in their lived realities, which are often socially and systemically produced and are the result of inadequate relational and structural resources (Yanicki et al., 2015).

An important role for CIs is to engage students to critically analyze and expand their awareness about social injustices that contribute to poor health. Students and nurses need to consider a lack of participation, recognition, and disadvantages for some groups may result from unequal power and opportunities. After analyzing these injustices, students will need to work with clients, communities, and populations to provide interventions aimed at influencing wider social policies and structures that determine health (Brunton et al., 2014). This may involve reforming social, political, and environmental conditions using social justice actions and considering upstream approaches to health (CNA, 2017; Cohen & Gregory, 2009b; Kirkham & Browne, 2006; Reutter & Kushner, 2010). For example, the NCCDH (2015) makes a distinction between engaging students with downstream thinking approaches, such as participating in a food drive to assist in the provision of food supplies for underprivileged groups at the food bank, and implementing upstream actions, which include meeting, planning, and advocating with community members for a living wage with their local member of Parliament.

Student Group-Based Interventions

Many community projects are facilitated through student group-based activities using various stages of the nursing process, such as gathering information using multiple sources and methods, critically analyzing the information gathered, setting priorities, and developing and implementing nursing interventions. These student projects mimic the larger work done by some provincial and territorial community teams when they engage in community assessment, planning, interventions, and evaluation of an interventions or community activity. Some of these group projects are undertaken over several years, with student groups moving in and out of the process depending on the stage of the project (Quinn et al., 2019; Williams et al., 2016). Group projects can cause angst for some students with their evaluation of learning. Instead of receiving individual evaluations and grades, students are evaluated with a group mark. CIs can support student learning in group activities by addressing group process skills, as discussed later in the chapter under teaching and learning strategies. As well, it is important that CIs provide a means for peer evaluation and for individual input into the overall final course grading rubric. Successful grading rubrics for group activities often have both individual and group components (discussed under teaching and learning strategies). Group process skills such as articulating oneself, negotiating different perspectives, collaborating with others to complete a project, working with others who have different working styles, and providing feedback can be useful for many facets of nursing and provide the opportunity for students to work with others on a time-limited team activity.

Collaboration with Non-health-care Providers and Sectors (Intersectoral Collaboration)

With structural and systemic barriers in access to health, intersectoral collaboration is required to transform systems, address social conditions that constrain health, and reduce inequities (Schroeder et al., 2019). CIs are instrumental in facilitating students' access to providers and professionals from sectors other than health to address strategies for change. These sectors may include education, justice, social services, mental health services, and disability supports as examples. These projects should include collaboration with community members and intersectoral providers with shared decision-making. For example, students can partake in community assessment meetings with various government sectors and community members. Students can also participate in social action interventions that change conditions influencing health, such as planning, developing, and building a playground and adding a green space in a subsidized housing complex.

Conferences and Conference Settings

The CI has an important role in facilitating student seminars or conferences. This includes face-to-face facilitation with students or providing feedback on students' written reflections by pulling in the community health nursing practice standards, addressing ethical questions/issues in practice, and bringing awareness to students regarding concerns that are unfolding in the community or larger systems. These learning strategies also occur in acute care clinical settings, but in community-oriented settings the CI highlights and addresses the intersection of more abstract concepts and ideas (e.g., social equity, social justice, upstream thinking, intersectoral collaboration) in the learning experiences with clients. Therefore, the CI uses strong facilitation skills in these interactions with students.

CIs must meet their students where they are when providing clinical education. This is often in community-oriented sites where the instructor may need to negotiate for use of space. Space is often limited in community settings and may need to be shared with multiple community partners. For example, the CI may be able to locate space at a community centre, community health clinic, school boardroom, or refugee centre. Sometimes this space becomes unavailable when timelines are short. Negotiating for space lends itself to learning about adapting and working with constraints when doing activities and group work in community settings.

It is important for CIs to have regular check-in points with students while they are engaged in their community projects, either as a group or individually. These check-ins are essential to clarify roles, addressing safety issues, dealing with team conflicts, teaching team building skills, and providing clarification about the project. Some of these issues are covered later in the chapter under challenges and strategies. Sometimes the CIs might be meeting students in public areas such as local coffee shops or community sites, which do not allow for confidentiality and may not be appropriate venues for sharing private information about a project. The CI will need to impart to the students the importance of confidentiality by not using client names or locations and by destroying/shredding any notes or documents containing community member information. In addition, CIs should review with students the social media policies from their postsecondary institution and remind students that they need to obtain written permission before taking pictures of community members engaged in any group activities.

Long-Term Immersion and Time in Placement Associated with Nursing Career Choice

Several studies have surveyed student nurses about career choices after graduation. Results have shown that graduates would not pick a career in community health nursing after being exposed to traditional placement sites, such as a public health nursing office (Larsen et al., 2012). Other researchers concluded that students may be reluctant to choose community health nursing as a specialization post-graduation because of several factors that reduce their comfort with the role, including lack of immersion in clinical skills, requirement to work with a community and population focus, and limited time in clinical placements (Brown, 2017; Williams et al., 2016). It is important that educators design nursing programs that expose students to clinical experiences and competencies in the community throughout their nursing programs. As well, students are often aware of the roles of RNs only in hospital and primary care settings and not in community health. Introduction to these diverse roles and competencies early in the curriculum can expose students to the multiple specialization opportunities in nursing.

Documentation of Nursing Activities in Community Placements

Students who are placed in traditional community PHN settings will use the documentation system that is used by nurses and other health care providers. Most urban community health centres have moved to electronic records and use a data system for documenting their nursing care. Alternatively, community projects in community-oriented non-traditional settings may have no official documentation process. The student group will likely develop a report to highlight their community assessment, plan, intervention, and evaluation following the nursing process. This type of report is a common documentation method used in public health nursing practice. This report can then be shared with community stakeholders and is a record of the assessment and work done by the community clinical group. Other nursing student cohorts and community members can also use the report and build on areas over time. Some of the challenges encountered by nurses, and therefore students, in all community-based settings include inconsistent Wi-Fi or internet access in homes and community agencies. Other issues centre on protection of confidentiality and privacy of records while on home visits, at schools, and at other agencies or while documenting nursing care while in a public setting such as a coffee shop. Issues with security of clients' records have arisen when nurses store work laptops in car trunks during visits or activities. The CI will need to follow the documentation policies from their community health placement site and share and enforce these with their students.

Roles of Clinical Instructors

In community health clinical education, the roles of CIs include important differences from those in acute care. In many educational programs, the CI in community placements may be called a faculty advisor rather than a CI. To be consistent with the terms used in other chapters, CI is used in this discussion of CI roles. There is a dearth of evidence on the roles of CIs in community placements, hence common practices in clinical teaching are discussed. The three CI roles of clinical supervisor, mentor and coach, and collaborator are explored and their nuances in community placements are described.

Clinical Supervisor

Typically, the clinical supervisor role in community placements has distinct differences from clinical supervision in acute care placements. Esteves et al. (2019) described clinical supervision as distinguished by nurses who are educators in postsecondary institutions and nurses who work in health care organizations. The nuance in clinical supervision in non-traditional community placements is that one nurse is responsible for the role of clinical supervisor and practitioner. Whereas in traditional health care placements such as acute care settings, clinical supervision is most often shared by the CI and the RN preceptor. In addition, Steffy (2019) conducted a study on how community health clinical experiences guide students in seeking a nursing role in community health nursing. The study found that clinical supervision and engagement by the CI during the placement enhances student learning (Steffy, 2019). Examples of how CIs are engaged in placements are described further in the section under teaching and learning strategies.

Another distinction in clinical supervision in non-traditional community placements is that the CI often provides an indirect model of supervision compared to direct supervision of individuals or groups of students in RN preceptor placements in the acute health sector. The focus in the discussion in this chapter is on indirect supervision in non-traditional community placements.

Indirect supervision means sporadic face-to-face (or distance) contact with a student group in non-RN and non-traditional community placements. Examples of face-to-face time with the students are conferences/praxis sessions or seminars and engagement with student groups in activities with their client population or key stakeholders, which all provide opportunities for clinical supervision (Babenko-Mould et al., 2016). CIs are typically not present for all clinical placement hours; hence, face-to-face time with students is only one part of the clinical evaluation. CIs are usually assigned a group of 8 to 12 students for an academic term. These students are then assigned to different community placement sites, each of which could range from two to six students, depending on the placement's capacity. The CI could be evaluating students in multiple placement sites. CIs assess student performance as a group and as individuals. CIs also use multiple evaluation strategies to grade students on activities they cannot directly observe. Of importance to curriculum developers for community health clinical placement is the inclusion of formative evaluation methods for both individual and group learning activities and individual summative evaluation processes to determine grades.

As noted, one CI may have students at several different placement sites. Therefore, CIs will often travel from one placement site to another to connect with students on the assigned clinical days (Valaitis et al., 2008). CIs usually hold an onsite conference with each student group lasting at least one hour. These conferences can take place at various locations, including the placement site, an alternative location in the community, or on campus. Student placement clinical hours vary across Canada and can range from 6 to 24 hours per week per term, depending on the specific educational program course requirements.

The non-RN community preceptor/community adviser is a key contact for the student group and liaises with the CI. They assist students to understand the community placement service mandate, vision, agency programs, and client population. They guide students to navigate the resources and assist them to network with community members (Babenko-Mould et al., 2016). They often provide feedback on the student groups' activities and on any student issues associated with these activities. The non-RN community preceptor may have some involvement in evaluation of student clinical performance, and they may meet regularly with the CI and with students to discuss activities (Cohen & Gregory, 2009a).

For CIs to provide effective indirect supervision, building on the roles described previously, they require knowledge of group dynamics and effective group facilitation skills, understanding and assessment of learning styles for each student in the group, and strategies to increase student engagement in group work. In addition to fulfillig the dual roles noted previously, CIs need to meet the CASN guidelines (2010) for faculty adviser/CIs, including current practice knowledge related to community and public health nursing, practice knowledge of the CCHN standards of practice (2019), knowledge regarding primary health care principles (CASN, 2014; World Health Organization [WHO], 1978) and CASN entry-to-practice PHN competencies.

Further, CIs in community placements focus on essential relational and decision-making skills rather than on teaching psychomotor skills or tasks in a well-supervised setting such as in an acute care learning environment (Ezhova et al., 2020; Feather et al., 2017). These skills include analysis of community and population needs, program planning and implementation, autonomous decision-making in the community placement while working with clients and community partners, advocacy, and communication with stakeholders to address care needs of clients and population groups (CASN, 2014). In community placements, CIs supervise clinical performance using their jurisdictional entry-level regulatory competencies, PHN competencies, and entry-level CCHN standards of practice (CASN, 2014; CHNC, 2019), in conjunction with their postsecondary institution's program philosophy and curriculum concepts. Student performance is assessed using the standards of practice, including the following:

- Prevention
- Health promotion
- Health maintenance
- Restoration and palliation
- Professional relationships
- Capacity building
- Health equity
- Evidence-informed practice
- Professional responsibility and accountability (CHNC, 2019)

The PHN knowledge, skills, and attitudes (competencies) include the following:

- Public health nursing sciences in nursing practice
- Population and community health assessment and analysis
- Population health planning, implementation, and evaluation
- Partnership, collaboration, and advocacy
- Communication in public health nursing (CASN, 2014)

Student Evaluation

A remedial plan for a student not meeting course objectives, or for a failing student in a community placement, is complex. The CI needs to assess the student's performance at an individual level separate from the group context. Formative assessment of performance can come from multiple sources such as these:
- Confidential peer feedback or observed behaviour in group performance (e.g., lack of engagement or not being a team player)
- Evidence of lack of professional responsibility with matters of punctuality (e.g., consistently late submission of course assignments or learning activities)
- Issues with attendance (e.g., consistently late or leaving early for placements)
- Community preceptor feedback about performance in placement (e.g., inappropriate language used with the client population or inappropriate attitudes displayed)
- Lack of conceptual understanding and application of theory in assignment or learning activities and conference discussions (e.g., lack of preparation and insufficient insight regarding community health concepts and approaches)
- Lack of clinical reasoning and judgement skills (e.g., insufficient gathering of information using multiple sources and methods, difficulty with priority setting in collaboration with client population, superficial interpretations, inadequate consideration of evidence information interventions)

When considering whether the student is practising safely, information from these multiple sources needs to be considered. When all or many of these areas for improvement are identified, the CI needs to meet with the student to discuss each concern. CIs need to be familiar with institutional expectations for students not meeting course expectations and work collaboratively with other faculty members accountable for the course. A sample remedial plan is described in Chapter 7.

Mentor and Coach

Like CIs in acute care placements, CIs in community placements are mentors and coaches (Brown, 2017). Meeley (2021) described role modelling in a mentor role as a powerful teaching tool in the community setting. As noted previously, the uniqueness of the CI role in community nursing is that the CI may be the only RN in contact with students in an indirect supervision model. Hence, CIs need to have current community and public health nursing practice experience to mentor students and an astute ability to coach students in practice development in an indirect supervised group learning model.

One example of mentoring students in a community health nursing practicum course can occur when students come to the course with no prior experience in caring for a client that is a community or population. A CI who is grounded in community and public health nursing practice mentors the students in their transition from a patient's illness narrative to a client community/population narrative by sharing their knowledge and expertise and by skilfully coaching students over the term with application of the "community health promotion model" (Yiu, 2020, p. 252) using the "community health nursing process" (pp. 265–267).

Another common mentoring and coaching example is assisting students to embrace and enact the nursing values of promotion of health and well-being and social justice, a responsibility in professional caring (CASN, 2014; CHNC, 2019; CNA, 2018). Although students have often heard about health promotion and social justice before taking the community health clinical course, CIs need to mentor students to expand the application and the "doing" of health promotion approaches beyond health teaching. For example, as the student group completes the community assessment in collaboration with the client population and sets priorities to address health inequities, the CI coaches them in advocating for strategies to promote health equity.

CIs also teach the nuances of leadership in community nursing practice by enhancing previous learning about the leadership role students bring with them to community nursing. Students in community placements develop their leadership skills in collaboration with others in their peer group and with other community members. For example, the student group may co-lead (with a principal, teacher, student council representative, or parent council member from a school community) a campaign on the theme of Turn off the Screen Week. The CI, using their practice knowledge, mentors the student group in this new perspective of leadership as a student team and coaches them to enable the client population to lead in planning and implementing the campaign.

Collaborator

The CI practices as a collaborator using their practice expertise in partnership building, one of the entry-level PHN competencies. CIs meet with their community placement student group in onsite conferences or praxis sessions, and these interactions may include community members who help to co-plan health promotion activities. Through CI role modelling, a collaborative dynamic partnership involving the CI, student team, and community members can be established. Students may develop the art of partnership, collaboration, and advocacy, which are not only PHN competencies (CASN, 2014), but also illustrate the primary health care principle of public participation (Lind & Baptiste, 2020; WHO, 1978).

Alexander (2020) noted that when CIs meet with students and their community partners to collaboratively plan and develop health promotion activities, they also facilitate community-academic partnerships. In addition, Valaitis et al. (2008), over a decade ago, highlighted that community academic partnerships fostered by CIs strengthen community health nursing educational experiences and are included as a criterion in the CASN (2010) guidelines for quality community health nursing placements. Ezhova et al. (2020) further described this co-working model of a teacher as an "experiential academic." The CI's professional skills in partnership building further illuminates the expected practice and competence of the CIs community health nursing expertise.

Through strengthening the community-academic partnership, the CI in a collaborator role contributes to building relationships with service providers and helps to pave the way for future community placement opportunities. With established professional relationships, over time, CIs recognize and identify quality community clinical learning opportunities that meet placement guidelines (CASN, 2010). These established relationships between academia and community are particularly important as the quality of available community placement opportunities continues to decline.

In the various roles described, the CIs use an array of teaching and learning strategies to support student achievement in community placements. The following section focuses on these strategies.

Teaching and Learning Strategies

An important consideration related to teaching strategies for CIs in community-oriented placements is recognizing what knowledge, skills, and attitudes related to community practice students bring with them to this new setting. Clinical courses in Canadian universities are situated across all four years of the program of study. More commonly, given the complexity of community and public health, clinical courses in community nursing education are situated in the last years of the BSN/BN program. Each community health clinical course has a course manual or syllabus outlining the course learning outcomes, expectations, required readings, and assessment and evaluation methods. In community placements, the details of community health promotion activities may be unknown until the students and faculty are involved with the client population and key stakeholders and determine their needs. Therefore, CIs work with students and placement sites to develop appropriate health promotion activities that are essential learning strategies.

Develop a Lesson Plan

As noted in Chapter 3, the lesson plan is a roadmap to assist students to achieve learning goals and indicates strategies for achieving those goals. In community placements, CIs need to help students make the shift from a structured hospital learning environment to a non-structured or minimally structured community setting. Also, students need to be guided to make the shift from immediate observations of change in a patient situation to a gradual, slow progression of change over time with a community as the client. An example of a slow progressive change is reduction of illness or injury in a specific population that may take months or years to be observable or measurable. A Gantt chart (see Figure 6.1) is a visual representation that enables students to see their progress related to learning outcomes over the academic term. When planning learning activities, the CI needs to consider how the theoretical assignments relate to clinical activities so that students make the connections between theory and community health nursing practice when achieving the learning outcomes. A review of previous learning and introduction of new relevant concepts are important strategies CI use with students before the first community placement visit.

Figure 6.1 *Sample Gantt Chart of Clinical Activities in a Community Placement over the Term Mapped to Course Learning Outcomes (CLOs) and Tanner's Model of Clinical Reasoning and Judgement (Community Health Nursing Process)*

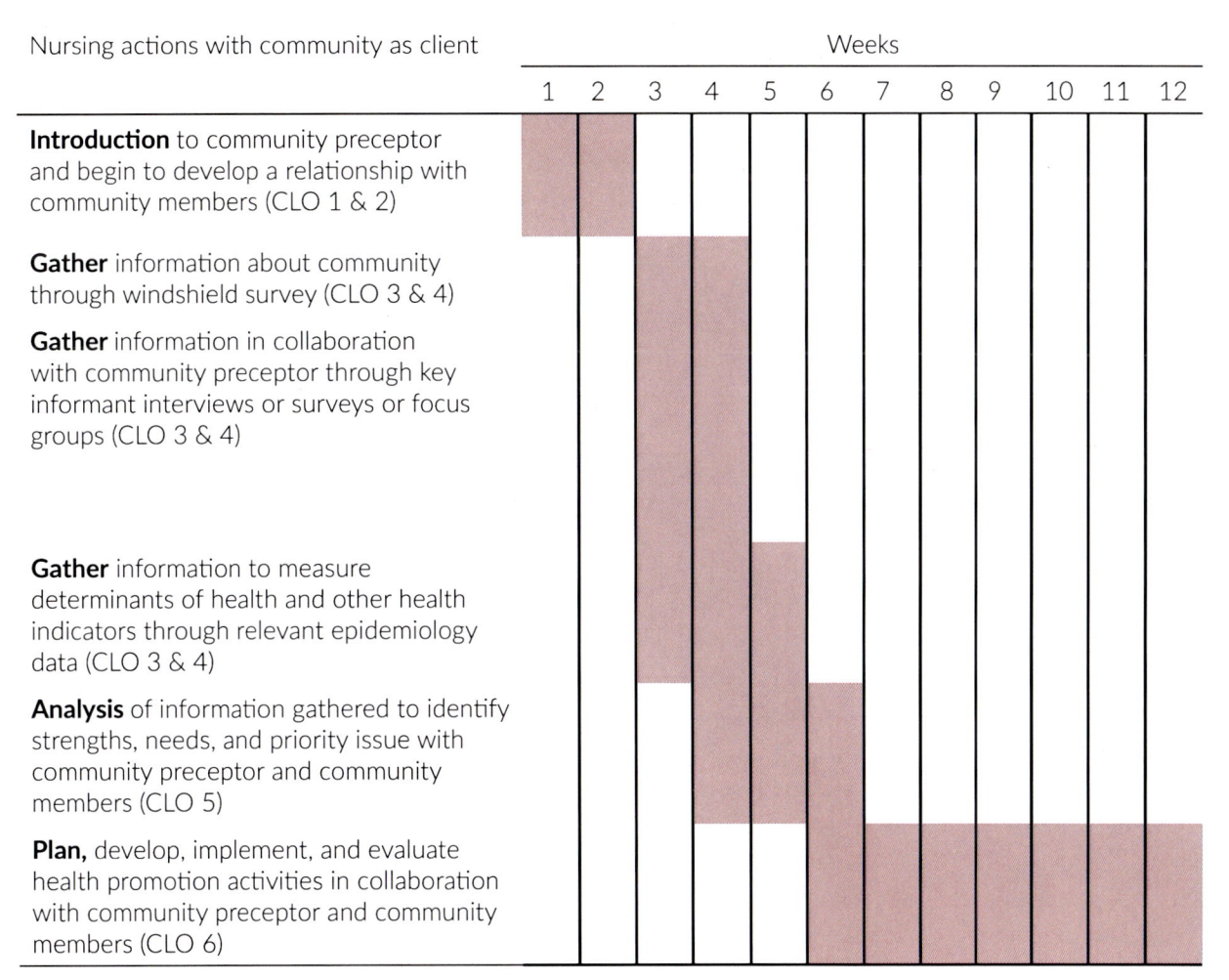

Nursing actions with community as client	Weeks 1–12
Introduction to community preceptor and begin to develop a relationship with community members (CLO 1 & 2)	Weeks 1–2
Gather information about community through windshield survey (CLO 3 & 4)	Weeks 3–5
Gather information in collaboration with community preceptor through key informant interviews or surveys or focus groups (CLO 3 & 4)	Weeks 3–5
Gather information to measure determinants of health and other health indicators through relevant epidemiology data (CLO 3 & 4)	Weeks 5–6
Analysis of information gathered to identify strengths, needs, and priority issue with community preceptor and community members (CLO 5)	Weeks 6–7
Plan, develop, implement, and evaluate health promotion activities in collaboration with community preceptor and community members (CLO 6)	Weeks 7–12

Source: Based in part on Tanner's model of clinical reasoning and judgement (2006).

Orient Students to Community Placement and PHN Practice

At the beginning of their clinical experience, students need to become familiar with a "typical" day in the life of a community and public health nurse. CIs can assist students to conceptualize the role of the nurse and guide them to the introduction of an autonomous practice (Williams et al., 2016). Using video clips, interviewing a CHN, shadowing a CHN, storytelling by CIs about their practice experiences, and using case studies are useful strategies to help students to become familiar with CHN practice. Shadowing a CHN depends on the CHN's availability. For example, if a CHN is involved with a school, or any of the potential placements noted previously, shadowing can be a meaningful learning experience as students observe or participate with the CHN in health promotion activities.

Students also need to become familiar with the layout of the placement site. Scavenger hunts or a team-based interactive exercise in which students gather information about the placement site, such as the mission, vision, programs, services, and so on, are examples of orientation activities that also cultivate teamwork skills. Small student groups can complete these activities using electronic sources and subsequently share their learning with other groups.

Entering the Community

Role-playing is a great teaching strategy to assist students to feel comfortable interacting with the client population before entering the placement site. Since students are strangers to the members of the community, a non-threatening informal interaction with the client population such as "hanging around" or going for coffee with clients can reduce feelings of fear and threat and build trust and rapport (Vollman, 2017). For example, if the students are at a homeless shelter, they can begin by saying hi, introducing themselves (wearing street clothes), initiate casual and non-health conversations, being present, listening, and letting people initiate interactions. The CIs role is to negotiate with the community preceptor for the first visit with students, which could be a triad meeting to discuss course and agency expectations and plans for communication. The community preceptor can give a tour of the site, which helps students to become familiar with the setting and reduces anxiety. This informal and trust-building time is important before beginning any community assessment. In addition, it is important for CIs to guide student teams in the most appropriate methods to use in a community assessment to minimize threat and discomfort among the client population while balancing the learning needs of students.

Support Self and Group Reflection

The following teaching strategy can enable students to develop competence in trauma-informed care, cultural safety approaches, and cultural humility with client populations in their community placement (Canadian Council for Registered Nurse Regulators [CCRNR], 2019; CHNC, 2019; McGibbon & Mbugua, 2020; Tisdale & McArthur, 2020). Many client populations encountered at community placements have experienced racism, including Black people, Indigenous people, and people of colour. In conference or praxis sessions, the CIs can facilitate a reflection process that examines personal and systemic biases. This activity also can be used to guide a discussion on historical and structural factors impacting the health of Indigenous Peoples and Indigenous knowledge or Indigenous rights (Tisdale & McArthur, 2020). For example, a self-reflection question could be, "Think about your own culture and what practices you cherish most, such as food, family, language, customs, and spirituality. Imagine that you are no longer able to connect with your culture. How would you feel? What would be some of the impacts on your life and well-being?" (Tisdale & McArthur, 2020, p. 422). Students engaged in group reflection would start with these questions: "What are the causes of disproportionately higher adverse health outcomes for Indigenous populations in Canada when compared to non-Indigenous populations? How can enforced geographic isolation contribute to issues related to the quality of life of Indigenous peoples? What are ways community and public health nurses can decolonize health promotion actions?" (Tisdale & McArthur, 2020, p. 422) "How would you go about gaining and demonstrating the skills and behaviours for culturally safe practice? How does culture influence health and illness within diverse communities? What roles do the social determinants of health and public policies play in the interplay of culture and health?" (McGibbon & Mbugua, 2020, p. 180).

Involve Students in Teaching Strategies

Student engagement is enhanced when they participate actively in learning. Ghasemi et al. (2020) found that when students, faculty, and community members actively shared learning opportunities with each other in a community partnership planning activity, students were motivated to be more engaged in new clinical learning environments. For example, students who were preparing to work with high school students on a vaping project met with high school students and their CI to share ideas. Then, through the team-based learning process, they developed a game to use with the high school students. To support evidence-informed content and quality practice-based learning, the CI reviewed the vaping project with the students before implementation.

Support Team-Based Learning

Community placements provide opportunities for team-based learning experiences. For example, Ghasemi et al. (2020) suggested CIs assist students to actualize the functioning of a PHN team (including selecting a student team leader) giving them the knowledge and skills to develop, implement, and evaluate a health promotion intervention in collaboration with the community members in their community placement. Ghasemi et al. (2020) found that team-based learning shapes student professional clinical behaviours, maximizes student participation in learning activities, develops active and deep learning, and strengthens teamwork performance, which in turn fosters student engagement in clinical settings. Refer to Chapter 2 for the CI role in supporting group dynamics.

Use Service-Learning Pedagogy

Non-traditional community placements are also sometimes described as service-learning experiences (Babenko-Mould et al., 2016; Dietrich-Leurer et al., 2011) and have been found to be a distinctive and engaging teaching strategy (Ghasemi et al., 2020). Service-learning is considered a partnership between academia and a community service agency. Students deliver nursing care and learn nursing competencies while working with communities to address their needs (Ghasemi et al., 2020; Stanley, 2013). Students in non-traditional placements work with client populations to achieve the population's health goals. Examples include a student nurse–led clinic in a refugee shelter (Thompson & Bucher, 2013) and the development of a proposal for a Tiny Homes affordable housing option accomplished by students in collaboration with the CI, a church community support program, and key community stakeholders.

The inclusion of critical social theory, a theoretical underpinning of community health nursing practice, assists students to broaden their understanding of complex social, economic, and political influences faced by equity-seeking groups. Critical social theory connects classroom content with real-world experience through service-learning (Stanley, 2013). The CI takes on the teaching role in this experiential pedagogy (McGahee et al., 2018; Schmidt et al., 2016).

Supporting Students to Enact Community and Public Health Nursing Practice

The CASN Public Health Nursing Teaching Strategies (2015) website offers many theoretical and clinical teaching strategies for CIs. A few clinical teaching strategies that illustrate "projects" students can be involved with are described below.
- Guide students through the application of the community health nursing process by using the "community health promotion model" (Yiu, 2020, p. 252), including a systematic community assessment, analysis, planning, interventions, and evaluation.
- Develop a health-related policy for an organization (e.g., non-use of vaping in high schools) in collaboration with students and staff (Callen et al., 2013).
- Plan a community health fair, in collaboration with a multicultural community service, that brings together multiple community health services to enable newcomers to become acquainted with the Canadian health care system.
- Develop, plan, implement, and evaluate a sustainable peer-led physical literacy intervention in an elementary school in collaboration with students, families, and school staff.

Challenges and Strategies in Community Clinical Education

Clinical educators and students encounter many challenges in community clinical settings. These can be related to implementation of curriculum goals and outcomes of community health nursing practice and the move beyond individual interventions to a broader focus on population and community-based health interventions. Strategies for managing these challenges are discussed below.

Collaborative Partnerships

Community clinical nursing education requires use of a collaborative/partnership model, which brings with it challenges because of the complexity of the issues and the multiple stakeholders involved. Further, community placement sites address conditions that influence the larger social determinants of health and lead to social inequities. Community-based students will likely work with clients and populations from diverse backgrounds and population groups. They require support from the CI in designing educational clinical experiences that move beyond a focus on individual behaviours and consider social issues that perpetuate poor health outcomes. Within collaborative partnerships, it is imperative that the CI and students build respectful relationships with community partners and agencies (Ezhova et al., 2020). Often these agency partnerships need to be renegotiated regularly and changes made as situations evolve (Williams et al., 2016). For example, COVID-19 restrictions encountered in 2020–2022 required CIs to use a variety of strategies to continue to work with community members to sustain student learning experiences. Strategies used included virtual meetings, simulation, and outdoor events.

Other examples of challenging (yet successful) collaborative partnerships include working with seniors, adults with mixed abilities, and preschoolers in a campus community gardening project to increase social inclusion and social connection, and decrease food insecurity (Jakubec et al., 2021); CIs partnering with a public health agency and families to provide nursing support for child growth and development, health assessments, and interventions through home visits and community programs to underserved families in a geographic community (Davis & Travers

Gustafson, 2015); and establishment of nurse-led clinics, in partnership with community agencies, to provide care to underserved populations by using a nursing model of care (Thompson & Bucher, 2013).

Sense of Autonomy, Self-Direction, and Role Ambiguity

Community placements are usually less structured, which brings students and CIs both challenges and opportunities. With less structure, loss of traditional acute care roles, use of non-traditional sites, and ambiguity about the role of nurses in health promotion, disease prevention, and population health planning, students may experience lack of role clarity (Callen et al., 2013; Ezhova et al., 2020; Pijl-Zieber & Kalischuk, 2011). CIs need to reinforce the roles of CHNs and develop realistic and feasible objectives for students regarding community work and course timelines when engaging with a community project or issue. CIs can remind students they have an opportunity to work with clients to influence barriers and facilitators to health at an earlier stage on the health spectrum. Students should also be encouraged to move beyond a focus on health education and individual behavioural intervention and towards upstream approaches that address sustainability and feasibility to enact changes in health and access to health (Schroeder et al., 2019). Students may also use their leadership, communication, decision-making, critical thinking and reasoning, and collaborative skills to partner with other providers and systems to enact change.

CIs need to help students become self-directed and clarify role ambiguity to achieve a sense of autonomy. Strategies to achieve this include activities that reinforce how to influence and enact health changes by meeting with community partners, facilitating participation from community members, informing and advocating for social and economic policies that impact health, analyzing current policies for their impacts on health, developing healthy public policy briefs, conducting nursing research on health reform measures, and transmitting knowledge translation strategies on system reform (Falk-Rafael & Betker, 2012; Rozendo et al., 2017; Reutter & Kushner, 2010).

Safety

While practicing in community settings, and facilitating population-based strategies, students are interacting with populations in unfamiliar geographic areas where they may be unsupervised by a clinical faculty member. Some geographic areas may provide services to underserved or hard to reach populations in urban or rural areas where there is little infrastructure and support. In addition, some locations may have higher crime or illegal drug use, have poor lighting, be geographically isolated, have deteriorating homes and apartment buildings, and involve hostile pets. CIs need to consider safety of students in all settings, including homes and shelters, schools, community clinics, refugee placement centres, worksites, and so on. It is important for CIs to outline potential risks and provide some safety guidelines (Maneval & Kurz, 2016). Safety strategies include recording where the student will be working and having a contact number so the CI can locate the student as necessary, planning for accessing emergency assistance, providing contact numbers, having students work in pairs or groups, ensuring students carry a cellphone, and asking clients to remove weapons, pets, and tobacco or other drugs before the student arrives in the home or setting. Environmental management also needs to be reviewed with students. Environmental management includes access to appropriate and reliable transportation to community sites such as well-maintained vehicles or public transit, accurate maps, awareness of travel times and parking availability, and considerations related to inclement weather and poor driving conditions (Beaver, 2014; Maneval & Kurz, 2016). CIs should follow policies for reporting incidents developed by the postsecondary institution.

Time Limitations and Course Outcomes

Community health nursing clinical courses are time limited because of the nature of the academic calendar. This can limit the time available to build relationships with community partners and agencies and time available to experience changes in health status (Diem & Moyer, 2009; Ezeonwu et al., 2014). Community stakeholders may be reluctant to invest in an academic partnership if these timelines are not worthy of the time and energy invested by partners (Ezeonwu et al., 2014; Williams et al., 2016). The CI must consider the constraints of these timelines and design short- and long-term course objectives and goals that are realistic for both students and community partners. This may mean designing different phases of a community social action project that students in different cohorts can move in and out of over several years. As an example, in the community-oriented campus garden with people of mixed abilities, preschoolers, and seniors, student cohorts focused on different phases of the project over time (Jakubec et al., 2021). Other academic programs have designed community health nursing clinical opportunities in which the same students work on the project over several years (Kruger et al., 2010; Quinn et al., 2019). Students can also be exposed to a variety of community-oriented experiences such as service learning and working with different populations throughout their nursing programs to develop clinical skills when working on community projects in different settings (Ezeonwu et al., 2014).

Evaluation Considerations

It can be challenging to evaluate student learning related to community-oriented competencies and concepts such as advocacy and social justice (Ezhova et al., 2020; Hanks, 2013). A public health intervention tool developed by Keller et al. (2004) provides measurable interventions that were tested by students in a school setting (Schaffer et al., 2016) and with physical activity and an ecological project (Olsen et al., 2017). Outcomes evaluated could include student growth through working with community members over a sustained period using leadership, engagement, negotiation, and group skills. Student work can also be evaluated with markers such as assessing community needs, employing research evidence, and knowledge translation strategies using social marketing tools to disseminate these interventions with infographics, posters, and videos. CIs can seek feedback from community members and students about community project interventions. This can include interviewing community members who were involved in projects and completing pre/post surveys with community members who participated in an intervention or used knowledge translation strategies (Quinn et al., 2019). Finally, students can contribute to evaluation of their own work using public health nursing competencies (Thompson & Bucher, 2013).

Summary

Practice-based learning in community, often non-traditional, placement settings is unique and complex for CIs and students. From a historical perspective, community and public health nursing has existed in the generalist preparation of a baccalaureate RN for over a century. The community clinical experience informs students' career choice. Characteristics of community nursing clinical education include new perspectives related to client and client-centred approaches; use of community and public health frameworks and standards to guide student group-based community health nursing processes; and working towards health equity actions in collaboration with the client as individual, family, community, population, and system and through partnerships with non-health-care providers and sectors. Other characteristics of the learning context include teaching and learning in varied conference settings and an expanded understanding of nursing documentation through report writing.

An effective CI is grounded in practice knowledge of community and public health nursing. The CI often integrates both educator and practitioner roles in these non-traditional and non-RN preceptor community placements. In addition, the CI role relates to indirect clinical supervision (being a mentor, coach, and collaborator), using multiple teaching and learning strategies, and managing challenges like collaborative partnerships, role ambiguity, safety, and time limitations.

Conclusion

A CI with strong experiential knowledge in community and public health is essential to effectively teach student groups expected practices and associated knowledge, skills, and attitudes for community health nursing practice, especially in non-traditional placements. CIs need to be grounded in the use of innovative collaborative teaching and learning strategies. They must also be able to espouse the tenets of client-centred, strength-based, and evidence-informed community and public health nursing practice to promote, protect, and preserve the health of individuals, families, groups, communities, populations, and systems to assist students to build their capacity to achieve entry-level competencies for nursing.

References

Alexander, G. K. (2020). Supporting food literacy among school and adolescents: Undergraduate students apply public health nursing principles in clinical practice. *Journal of Professional Nursing, 36*, 616–624. https://doi.org/10.1016/j.profnurs.2020.08.018

Babenko-Mould, Y., Ferguson, K., & Atthill, S. (2016). Neighbourhood as community: A qualitative descriptive study of nursing students' experiences of community health nursing. *Nurse Education in Practice, 17*, 223–228. https://doi.org/10.1016/j.nepr.2016.02.002

Beaver, D. (2014). Visiting nurse service and home healthcare visitation safety. *Journal of Healthcare Protection Management: Publication of the International Association for Hospital Security, 30*(2), 107–116. PMID: 25181799

Bekemeier, B., & Butterfield, P. (2005). Unreconciled inconsistencies: A critical review of the concept of social justice in 3 national nursing documents. *Advances in Nursing Science, 28*(2), 152–162. https://doi.org/10.1097/00012272-200504000-00007

Bekemeier, B., Walker Linderman, T., Kneipp, S., & Zahner, S. J. (2015). Updating the definition and role of public health nursing to advance and guide the specialty. *Public Health Nursing, 32*(1), 50–57. https://doi.org/10.1111/phn.12157

Bourque Bearskin, R. (2011). A critical lens on culture in nursing practice. *Nursing Ethics, 18*(4), 548–559. https://doi.org/10.1177/0969733011408048

Brown, C. (2017). Linking public health nursing competencies and service-learning in a global setting. *Public Health Nursing, 34*, 485–492. https://doi.org/10.1111/phn.12330

Brunton, G., O'Mara-Eves, A., & Thomas, J. (2014). The 'active ingredients' for successful community engagement with disadvantaged expectant and new mothers: A qualitative comparative analysis. *Journal of Advanced Nursing, 70*, 2847–2860. https://doi.org/10.1111/jan.12441

Callen, B., Smith, C., Joyce, B., Lutz, J., Brown-Schott, N., & Block, D. (2013). Teaching/Learning strategies for the essential of baccalaureate nursing education for entry-level community/public health nursing. *Public Health Nursing, 30*(6), 537–547. https://doi.org/10.111/phn.12033

Canadian Association of Schools of Nursing. (2010). *Guidelines for quality community health nursing clinical placements for baccalaureate nursing students.* https://casn.ca/wp-content/uploads/2014/12/CPGuidelinesFinalMarch.pdf

Canadian Association of Schools of Nursing. (2014). *Entry-to-practice public health nursing competencies for undergraduate nursing education.* https://casn.ca/wp-content/uploads/2014/12/FINALpublichealthcompeENforweb.pdf

Canadian Association of Schools of Nursing. (2015). *Public health nursing teaching strategies.* http://publichealth.casn.ca/

Canadian Council for Registered Nurse Regulators. (2019). *Entry-level competencies for the practice of registered nurses.* https://www.ccrnr.ca/assets/ccrnr-rn-entry-level-competencies---2019.pdf

Canadian Nursing Association. (2015). *Primary health care position statement.* https://hl-prod-ca-oc-download.s3-ca-central-1.amazonaws.com/CNA/2f975e7e-4a40-45ca-863c-5ebf0a138d5e/UploadedImages/documents/Primary_health_care_position_statement.pdf

Canadian Nursing Association. (2017). *Code of ethics.* https://hl-prod-ca-oc-download.s3-ca-central-1.amazonaws.com/CNA/2f975e7e-4a40-45ca-863c-5ebf0a138d5e/UploadedImages/documents/Code_of_Ethics_2017_Edition_Secure_Interactive.pdf

Cohen, B. E., & Gregory, D. (2009a). Community health clinical education in Canada: Part 1, "state of the art." *International Journal of Nursing Education Scholarship, 6*(1), 1–15. https://doi.org/10.2202/1548-923X.1637

Cohen, B. E., & Gregory, D. (2009b). Community health clinical education in Canada: Part 2, developing competencies to address social justice, equity, and the social determinants of health. *International Journal of Nursing Education Scholarship, 6*(2), 1–17. https://doi.org/10.2202/1548-923X.1638

Community Health Nurses of Canada. (2019). *Canadian community health nursing professional practice model & standards of practice.* https://www.chnc.ca/en/standards-of-practice

Davis, R. A., & Travers Gustafson, D. (2015). Academic-practice partnership in public health nursing: Working with families in a village-based collaboration. *Public Health Nursing, 32*, 327–338. https://doi.org/10.1111/phn.12135

Diem, E., & Moyer, A. (2009). Development and testing of tools to evaluate public health nursing clinical education at the baccalaureate level. *Public Health Nursing, 27*(3), 285–293. https://doi.org/10.1111/j.1525-1446.2010.00855.x

Dietrich-Leurer, M. A., Meagher-Stewart, D., Cohen, B., Seaman, P. M., Granger, M., & Pattullo, H. (2011). Developing guidelines for quality community health nursing clinical placements for baccalaureate nursing students. *International Journal of Nursing Education Scholarship, 8*(1), 1–13. https://doi.org/10.2202/1548-923X.2297

Duncan, S., Scaia, M. R., & Boschema, G. (2020). "100 years of university nursing education": The significance of a baccalaureate nursing degree and its public health origins for nursing now. *Quality Advancement in Nursing Education, 6*(2), 1–15. https://doi.org/10.17483/2368-6669.1248

Esteves, L. S. F., Cunha, I. C. K. O., Bohomol, E., & Santos, M. R. (2019). Clinical supervision and preceptorship/tutorship: Contributions to the supervised curricular internship in nursing education. *Revista Brasileira de Enfermagem, 72*(6), 1730–1735. http://dx.doi.org/10.1590/0034-7167-2018-0786

Ezeonwu, M., Berkowitz, B., & Vlasses, F. R. (2014). Using an academic-community partnership model and blended learning to advance community health nursing pedagogy. *Public Health Nursing, 31*(3), 272–280. https://doi.org/10.1111/phn.12060

Ezhova, I., Sayer, L., Newland, R., Davis, N., McLetchie-Holder, S., Burrows, P., Middleton, L., & Malone, M. E. (2020). Models and frameworks that enable nurses to develop their public health practice: A scoping study. *Journal of Clinical Nursing, 29*(13–14), 2150–2160. https://doi.org/10.1111/jocn.15267

Falk-Rafael, A., & Betker, C. (2012). Witnessing social injustice downstream and advocating for health equity upstream: "The trombone slide" of nursing. *Advances in Nursing Science, 35*, 98–112. https://doi.org/10.1097/ANS.0b013e31824fe70f

Feather, J., Carter, N., Valaitis, R., & Kirkpatrick, K. (2017). A narrative evaluation of a community-based nurse navigation role in an urban at-risk community. *Journal of Advanced Nursing, 73*, 2997–3006. https://doi.org/10.1111/jan.13355

Fornoda, C., Baptiste D. L., Reinholdt, M. M., & Ousman, K. (2016). Cultural humility: A concept analysis. *Journal of Transcultural Nursing, 27*, 210–217. https://doi.org/10.1177/1043659615592677

Ghasemi, M. R., Moonaghi, H. K., & Heydan, A. (2020). Strategies for sustaining and enhancing nursing students' engagement in academic and clinical settings: A narrative review. *Korean Journal of Medical Education, 32*(2), 103–117. https://doi.org/10.3946/kjme.2020.159

Gottlieb, L. (2013). *Strength-based nursing care: Health and healing for person and family.* Springer Publishing Company.

Hanks, R. G. (2013). Social advocacy: A call for nursing action. *Pastoral Psychology, 62*, 163–173. https://doi.org/10.1007/s11089-011-0404-1

Health Protection and Promotion Act, RSO 1990, c. H.7. https://www.ontario.ca/laws/statute/90h07

Jakubec, S. L., Szabo, J., Gleeson, J., Currie, G., & Flessati, S. (2021). Planting seeds of community-engaged pedagogy: Community health nursing practice in an intergenerational campus-community gardening program. *Nurse Education in Practice, 51*, 102980, 1–7. https://doi.org/10.1016/j.nepr.2021.102980

Keller, L. O., Strohschein, S., Schaffer, M. A., & Lia-Hoagberg, B. (2004). Population-based public health interventions: Innovations in practice, teaching, and management. (Part II). *Public Health Nursing, 21*, 469–487. https://doi.org/10.1111/j.0737-1209.2004.21510.x

Kirkham, S. R., & Browne, A. (2006). Toward a critical theoretical interpretation of social justice discourses in nursing. *Advances in Nursing Science, 29*(4), 324–339.

Kruger, B. J., Roush, C., Olinzock, B. J., & Bloom, K. (2010). Engaging nursing students in a long-term relationship with a home-base community. *Journal of Nursing Education, 49*(1), 10–16. https://doi.org/10.3928/01484834-20090828-07

Larsen, R., Reif, L., & Frauendienst, R. (2012). Baccalaureate nursing students' intention to choose a public health career. *Public Health Nursing, 29*(5), 424–432. https://doi.org/10.1111/j.1525-1446.2012.01031

Lathrop, B. (2013). Nursing leadership in addressing the social determinants of health. *Policy, Politics, & Nursing Practice, 14*, 41–47. https://doi.org/10.1177/1527154413489887

Lind, C., & Baptiste, L. (2020). Health Promotion. In L. L. Stamler, L. Yiu, A. Dosani, J. Etowa, & C. van Daalen-Smith (Eds.), *Community health nursing: A Canadian perspective* (5th ed., pp. 137–167). Pearson.

Maneval, R. E., & Kurz, J. (2016). "Nursing students assaulted": Considering student safety in community-focused experiences. *Journal of Professional Nursing, 32*(3), 246–251. https://doi.org/10.1016/j.profnurs.2015.11.001

McGahee, T., Bravo, M., Simmons, L., & Reid, T. (2018). Nursing students and service learning: Research from a symbiotic community partnership with local schools and special Olympics. *Nurse Educator, 43*(4), 215–218. https://doi.org/10.1097/NNE.0000000000000445

McGibbon, E., & Mbugua, J. (2020). Race, culture, and health. In. L. L. Stamler, L. Yiu, A. Dosani, J. Etowa, & C. van Daalen-Smith (Eds.), *Community health nursing: A Canadian perspective* (5th ed., pp. 168–182). Pearson.

Meeley, N. G. (2021). Undergraduate student nurses' experiences of their community placements. *Nurse Education Today, 106*, 105054. https://doi.org/10.1016/j.nedt.2021.105054

National Collaborating Centre for Determinants of Health. (2015). *Let's talk: Advocacy and health equity*. National Collaborating Centre for Determinants of Health. http://nccdh.ca/images/uploads/comments/Advocacy_EN.pdf

National Collaborating Centre for Determinants of Health. (2020a). *Let's talk: Values and health equity*. https://nccdh.ca/resources/entry/lets-talk-values-and-health-equity

National Collaborating Centre for Determinants of Health. (2020b). *Let's talk: Ethical foundations of health equity*. https://nccdh.ca/resources/entry/lets-talk-ethical-foundations-of-health-equity

Olsen, J. M., Baisch, M. J., & Monsen, K. A. (2017). Interpretation of ecological theory for physical activity with the Omaha System. *Public Health Nursing, 34*(1), 59–68. https://doi.org/10.1111/phn.12277

Phillips, G., & Schofield, R. (2020). Nursing roles, functions, and practice settings. In. L. L. Stamler, L. Yiu, A. Dosani, J. Etowa, & C. van Daalen-Smith (Eds.), *Community health nursing: A Canadian perspective* (5th ed., p. 40). Pearson.

Pijl-Zieber, E. M., & Kalischuk, R. G. (2011). Community health nursing practice education: Preparing the next generation. *International Journal of Nursing Education Scholarship, 8*(1), 1-13. https://hdl.handle.net/10133/5097

Pijl-Zieber, E. M., Barton, S., Awosoga, O., & Konkin, J. (2015). Disconnect in pedagogy and practice in community health nursing clinical experiences: Qualitative findings in a mixed method study. *Nurse Education Today, 35*, e43-e48. https://doi.org/10.1016/j.nedt.2015.08.012

Public Health Agency of Canada. (2017). *Framework for ethical deliberation and decision-making in public health a tool for public health practitioners, policy makers and decision makers.* https://www.canada.ca/content/dam/phac-aspc/documents/corporate/transparency/corporate-management-reporting/internal-audits/audit-reports/framework-ethical-deliberation-decision-making/pub-eng.pdf

Quinn, B. L., El Ghaziri, M., & Knight, M. (2019). Incorporating social justice, community partnerships, and student engagement in community health nursing courses. *Teaching and Learning in Nursing, 14*(3), 183-185. https://doi.org/10.1016/j.teln.2019.02.006

Reutter, L., & Kushner, K. E. (2010). Health equity through action on the social determinants of health: Taking up the challenge in nursing. *Nursing Inquiry, 17*(3), 269-280. https://doi.org/10.1111/j.1440-1800.2010.00500.x

Rozendo, C. A., Salas, A. S., & Cameron, B. (2017). A critical review of social and health inequalities in the nursing curriculum. *Nurse Education Today, 50*, 62-71. https://doi.org/10.1016/j.nedt.2016.12.006

Schaffer, M. A., Anderson, L. J., & Rising, S. (2016). Public health interventions for school nursing practice. *The Journal of School Nursing, 32*(3), 195-208. https://doi.org/10.1177/1059840515605361

Schmidt, S., George, M., & Bussey-Jone, J. (2016). Welcome to the neighborhood: Service learning to understand social determinants of health and promote local advocacy. *Diversity and Equality in Health Care, 13*(6), 389-390. https://diversityhealthcare.imedpub.com/welcome-to-the-neighborhood-service-learning-to-understand-of-social-determinants-of-healthand-promote-local-advocacy.php?aid=17441

Schroeder, K., Garcia, B., Phillips, R. S., & Lipman, T. H. (2019). Addressing social determinants of health through community engagement: An undergraduate nursing course. *Journal of Nursing Education, 58*(7), 423-426. https://doi.org/10.3928/01484834-20190614-07

Stanley, M. J. (2013). Teaching about vulnerable populations: Nursing students' experience in a homeless center. *Journal of Nursing Education, 52*(10), 585-588. https://doi.org/10.3928/01484834-20130913-03

Steffy, M. L. (2019). Community health learning experiences that influence RN to BSN students interests in community/public health nursing. *Public Health Nursing, 36*, 863-871. https://doi.org/10.1111/phn.12670

Tanner, C. (2006). Thinking like a nurse: A researched-based model of clinical judgment in nursing. *Journal of Nursing Education, 45*(6), 204-211. https://doi.org/10.3928/01484834-20060601-04

Thompson, C. W., & Bucher, J. A. (2013). Meeting baccalaureate public/ community health nursing education competencies in nurse-managed wellness centers. *Journal of Professional Nursing, 29*, 155-162. https://doi.org/10.1016/j.profnurs.2012.04.017

Tisdale, D., & McArthur, G. C. (2020). Indigenous health. In L. L. Stamler, L.Yiu, A. Dosani, J. Etowa, & C. van Daalen-Smith (Eds.), *Community health nursing: A Canadian perspective* (5th ed., pp. 406-425). Pearson.

Tunis, B. I. (1996). *In caps and gowns: The story of the school of graduate nurses at McGill University, 1920-1964.* McGill University Press.

Valaitis, R. K., Rajsic, C., Cohen, B., Stamler, L. L., Meagher-Stewart, D., & Froude, S. A. (2008). Preparing the community health nursing workforce: Internal and external enablers and challenges influencing undergraduate nursing education in Canada. *International Journal of Nursing Education Scholarship, 5*(10), 1-21. https://doi.

org/10.2202/1548-923X.1518

Van Doren, E. S., & Vander Werf, M. (2012). Developing nontraditional community health placements. *Journal of Nursing Education, 51*(1), 46–49. https://doi.org/10.3928/01484834-20111116-04

Vollman, A. (2017). Community assessment. In A. Vollman & S. Jackson (Eds.), *Canadian community as partner: Theory and multidisciplinary practice* (pp. 222–247). Wolters Kluwer/Lippincott Williams & Wilkins.

Vukic, A., & Dilworth, K. (2020). The history of community health nursing in Canada. In L. L. Stamler, L. Yiu, A. Dosani, J. Etowa, & C. van Daalen-Smith (Eds.), *Community health nursing: A Canadian perspective* (5th ed., p. 7). Pearson.

Williams, J. R., Halstead, V., & McKim Mitchell, E. (2016). Two models for public health nursing clinical education. *Public Health Nursing, 33*(3), 249–255. https://doi.org/10.1111/phn.12256

World Health Organization. (1978). *Primary health care.* https://www.who.int/health-topics/primary-health-care

Yanicki, S. M., Kushner, K. E., & Reutter, L. (2015). Social inclusion/exclusion as matters of social (in) justice: A call for nursing action. *Nursing Inquiry, 22*(2), 121–133. https://doi.org/10.1111/nin.12076

Yiu, L. (2020). Community nursing process. In L. L. Stamler, L. Yiu, A. Dosani, J. Etowa, &C. van Daalen-Smith (Eds.), *Community health nursing: A Canadian perspective* (5th ed., pp. 247–270). Pearson.

Acknowledgements: We would like to acknowledge Dr. Andrea Chircop, associate professor, Dalhousie University; Tanya Sanders, associate teaching professor, Thompson Rivers University; and Melissa Raby, sessional adjunct professor, Queen's University, for their critical review and contributions to this chapter.

CHAPTER 7

Assessing and Evaluating Students in the Clinical Setting

Karin Page-Cutrara

This chapter provides an overview of the clinical evaluation process that guides clinical instructors in the judgement of student's performance. An overview of this process, which includes its purpose, various ways in which the process can be established, supports for both the clinical instructor and the student, and the difference between formative and summative evaluation is presented. Strategies for supporting the student during the learning period, providing ongoing feedback, and communicating a final decision are emphasized.

Chapter Objectives

After completing the chapter, the reader will be able to
- differentiate between assessment and evaluation in clinical teaching
- outline the clinical evaluation process, including the purpose, components, and methods for supporting intended outcomes
- identify a variety of approaches to, and challenges with, formative evaluation of a student in the clinical practice environment
- describe approaches and tools for facilitating the summative evaluation of clinical performances

Introduction

A student's performance in the clinical setting can be a challenge to evaluate. For nurses that are new to a clinical instructor (CI) role, clinical evaluation can seem particularly daunting because of the judgement and finality of the decision-making that may be involved. For those nurses who have more experience in the teaching role, clinical evaluation may remain a challenge because of the nature of learning in dynamic clinical settings and the various and unique needs of students as learners.

The aim of clinical learning in a direct-care environment is for students to develop essential professional competencies for safe and ethical nursing practice. Competencies related to psychomotor skills, communication, application of nursing theoretical knowledge and related sciences, professional and leadership behaviours, ethical decision-making, and the use of research may be learned separately in classroom settings and are often applied through constructed case studies or scenarios. However, such competencies cannot be demonstrated fully in the classroom or the laboratory, and so the practice of nursing care must be supported and measured in the clinical setting. The application of these competencies in a live patient care environment requires the ability for students to not only integrate knowledge but also adapt and respond to unpredictable changes in health and health care systems. This dynamic nature of clinical education, essential as it is for new nurses to experience, contributes to the complexity of evaluating students' performance.

This chapter presents the complex nature of evaluation in the clinical setting. After a short background discussion of clinical evaluation, initial assessment of the student, personal learning plans and communication of outcomes are discussed as a foundation for clinical learning. The significance of formative feedback and how to deliver it will be presented, as well as methods for ongoing collection of performance data, and associated approaches for supporting remediation and progression planning. Summative evaluations, compared to formative feedback, are described, in addition to communication and documentation of the acquisition of learning outcomes in relation to prescribed expectations.

Background and Overview of Assessment and the Clinical Evaluation Process

In nursing education, demonstrated clinical performance has always been a significant component of a student's evaluation within the nursing education context. Student performance is a direct indicator for determining how safe and competent a student would be as a practising nurse. In Canada, the clinical teaching-learning unit for nursing student learning is like that offered by other health care professions' educational programs. Comprising small groups that are facilitated and supervised by a CI, or as a one-on-one preceptored experience, these unit structures are typical of how academic centres create teaching, supervisory, and evaluative supports for clinical learning. In fact, such traditional clinical learning structures are foundational to clinical learning across the globe (Leighton et al., 2021).

The structure of the teaching-learning unit, and the methods and tools for assessing and evaluating learning outcomes, contribute to the challenging nature of evaluation in clinical education. Research evidence and the state of the science relating to clinical evaluation in nursing tend to show that breadth but not depth is the main criterion in evaluation. While 50 years of research have addressed topics such as competence, measurement tools, teaching methods, grading processes, and clinical reasoning, few studies have built on previous work, resulting in a weak body of knowledge in the area of clinical evaluation (Lewallen & Van Horn, 2019). Furthermore, a systematic review of the literature conducted by Leighton and colleagues (2021) revealed that no sufficient evidence was found to support learning outcomes that could be attributed to current, traditional clinical education models or structures (i.e., group of students supervised by a CI or preceptor). This result creates serious concerns about the reliance on such models for the assessment and evaluation of students' clinical performance and continues to frame clinical education in nursing as a "relatively unsystematic apprenticeship process" (Gaba, 2004, p. i2).

Nevertheless, a student's clinical teaching-learning experience, led by a CI or preceptor, remains the standard. Regardless of the current challenges, understanding the traditional clinical evaluation process is vital before engaging in the education of students in the clinical setting.

In the context of nursing education, *clinical evaluation* can be described as part of the teaching-learning process whereby a judgement about a student's achievement of predetermined behavioural outcomes or standards is made, based on the collection and analysis of specific and multifaceted performance data that relate to the integration of cognitive, psychomotor, and affective knowledge in a direct-care environment (Lewallen & Van Horn, 2019; Oermann et al., 2022). Clinical evaluation seeks to articulate the extent to which a student has applied theoretical knowledge to the nursing practice environment.

Assessment and *evaluation* are two terms that are often used interchangeably. In the clinical evaluation process, the *assessment* of the student by the CI refers to collecting data about a student's acquired knowledge and level of performance. Assessment is aimed at determining learning gaps to be addressed and assists with planning relevant instructional activities (Oermann et al., 2022).

Evaluation is the process of making determinations about a student's performance. Evaluation, when compared to assessment, is differentiated primarily by *purpose* and is often separated into two activities. Formative evaluation is an ongoing activity that is diagnostic and, in this way, is comparable with assessment (Brookhart & Nitko, 2015). However, formative evaluation is feedback in relation to a standard and so is conducted to improve future performance; formative evaluation is an evaluation *for learning*. Sometimes referred to as midterm or mid-course clinical evaluations, formative evaluations may not necessarily include a mark and normally precede summative evaluations. Summative evaluation is a final determination or judgement of whether a student has achieved the specific clinical outcomes or competencies (Oermann et al., 2022). Summative evaluation is an evaluation *of learning* (see Figure 7.1).

Figure 7.1 *A Comparison of Formative and Summative Clinical Course Evaluation*

Formative evaluation	Summative evaluation
Improve future behaviours	Describe final performance
Ongoing activities	One-time activity
Diagnostic	Judgemental
Interim grade/not graded	Final grade
Occurs at mid-course	Occurs at end of course

The clinical evaluation process involves an initial assessment of the student, a formative evaluation, and a summative evaluation that culminates in a judgement of student performance in the clinical setting (see Figure 7.2). These components, guided by clinical course outcomes, are presented in the following sections.

Figure 7.2 *The Clinical Evaluation Process*

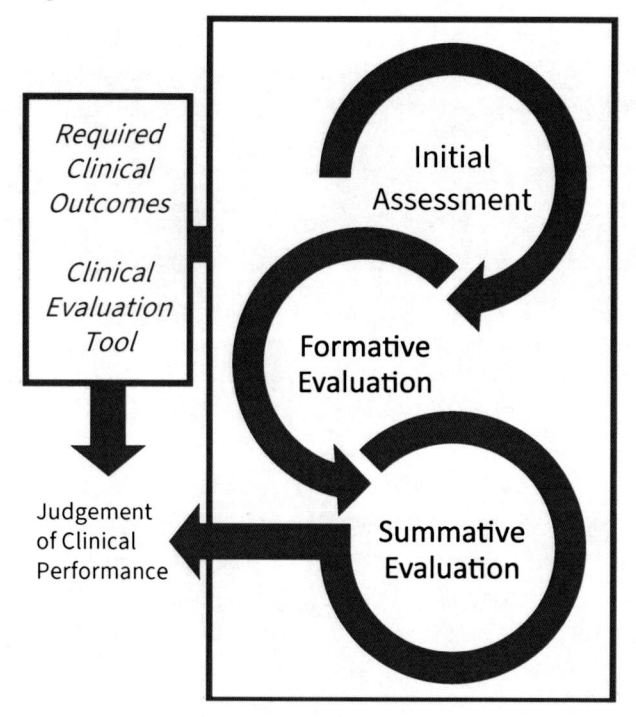

Initial Assessment of the Student

As noted earlier, assessment, which is different from evaluation, can be described as activities aimed at collecting information on current and prior knowledge and experiences in relation to a specific goal or outcome, and establishing what a student knows or understands about an aspect of nursing practice in relation to what is expected. This collection of information can occur through direct observation, student self-report, or peer feedback, and analysis may be further informed by additional available information. Assessment can therefore be either a discrete activity or an ongoing activity; often, ongoing assessment is associated with formative evaluation. In the clinical context, the purpose of student assessment is to understand the learner and their needs for understanding nursing practice in relation to a specific clinical course.

The initial assessment of students provides an essential foundation for the evaluation process. This first part of the clinical evaluation process starts when the CI is assigned to a student or group of students. The CI must approach clinical evaluation as a systematic and continual process aimed at providing timely, appropriate, and meaningful feedback that is both useful to the individual student and reflective of achievement of required outcomes of the course or program.

At the outset of a clinical course, the CI must seek to understand the unique learning needs of the assigned student or group of students to facilitate achievement of course outcomes. Oermann et al. (2022) outline five approaches to use when assessing students: identify outcomes, select appropriate assessment methods, meet students' needs, use multiple assessment methods, and recognize limitations of assessments. In terms of the initial assessment of students that supports evaluation in the clinical setting, CIs should consider similar activities as follows:

- Check biases, values, and assumptions
- Identify course outcomes to be achieved
- Conduct needs assessment using various resources
- Create plans for learning

While discussed in earlier chapters, these activities are presented here as they support the clinical evaluation process.

Examining Bias, Values, and Assumptions

Determination of a student's competence can be perceived as both objective and subjective. In fact, many resources clearly indicate that the process is more subjective than objective (Oermann & Gaberson, 2017; McGregor, 2007). The CI's values can influence evaluation of a student's performance.

Chapter 3 outlines different ways to become aware of bias when teaching. In terms of the clinical evaluation process, Fainstad et al. (2021) identified a three-step method for addressing cognitive bias in assessment:

- First, *name*, which involves a simple admission about the presence of inherent bias in assessment.
- Next, *reframe*, which involves rephrasing assessment language to shed light on the instructor's subjectivity.
- Last, *check-in*, which offers a chance to ensure student understanding and opens lines of bidirectional communication between the student and instructor.

Such approaches are useful in increasing instructor awareness of the existence and influence of unconscious bias.

Additionally, a CI's self-reflective stance in terms of any perceptions and pre-judgements for what makes a good nurse in a particular clinical setting, their previous teaching and evaluation experiences, and personal interpretations of competency or outcome requirements can help with reducing the extent to which bias may have an unfair effect on a student's evaluation. A student who is shy and who may not participate as actively as others in a post-conference discussion should not be judged as less competent or less engaged in other areas. Novice students placed in fast-paced acute clinical settings, who may not be able to make decisions or respond quickly, should not have the same expectations for their performance as more senior students that the CI has supervised in the past.

The characteristics of the CI, in terms of approachability and ability to communicate, significantly affect the nature of the evaluation process and the student's receptivity to (and response to) feedback. These instructor qualities were discussed in previous chapters. The ultimate requirement for the CI is to provide a judgement of a student's performance in a fair, non-threatening, and non-judgemental manner, free of perceived bias. Specific considerations for ethics of teaching and learning in the clinical environment are reviewed in a later chapter.

Identifying Course Outcomes and Requirements

It is essential, in the initial assessment of students and their learning needs, that the CI be familiar with the course outcomes and the required activities that support the achievement of those outcomes. The CI should be familiar with the theoretical knowledge that is delivered in a particular course. To accurately assess how students are positioned to learn, the anticipated outcomes must be clear and must be communicated to students. This communication ensures that the CI fully appreciates what is expected of the students and the knowledge requirements at a specific point in the program.

The expectations for rating students' performances should be well defined. During the clinical evaluation process, the CI observes performance, collects data. and compares them to intended outcomes to arrive at a judgement (Oermann & Gaberson, 2017). Additional expectations for meeting professional behavioural standards, or national or provincial or territorial competencies, should be highlighted if they are not articulated in the course outcomes. These expectations can include arriving on time or using a respectful tone in all communications.

Outcomes of students' clinical experiences are the result of all teaching-learning activities aimed at supporting practice-based performance and are what students are required to demonstrate at the end of a clinical course. Because of their importance to a students' success in a program and to their achievement of competence, outcomes of clinical experiences should be framed as clear objectives or competencies that specifically relate to the course goals. These typically include cognitive, psychomotor, and affective domains of learning. Expected outcomes must be communicated to students at the outset of the clinical course.

Students must be aware that they will be assessed in a variety of ways in the clinical setting. Cognitive skills that are evaluated relate to demonstration of critical thinking and problem-solving, clinical reasoning in the direct-care environment, and clinical judgements made by the students in relation to professional collaborations and the science-based nursing care provided (Baker, 2020). Psychomotor skills are evaluated in outcomes that reflect not only the efficiency, organization, and effectiveness of the physical care provided but also the physical aspects of therapeutic, intra- and interprofessional communication, such as speaking, non-verbal behaviours, and documentation. Evaluation of the affective domain is also shared, and performance outcomes such as respectful engagement with patients, cultural humility, ethical and compassionate provision of care, professional socialization and sense of independence, and commitment to professional growth and development are often included as performance outcomes.

Many programs include a predetermined number of clinical course hours for a student to attend in the clinical setting so that all students have a reasonable opportunity to demonstrate the course outcomes. There is much debate, and no conclusive evidence, that a specific number of hours is necessary to ensure competence; every program and its students are different. Programs may develop departmental policies that support students' attendance and completion of required clinical hours.

Assessing Students' Clinical Learning Needs

Typically, information about the course level (i.e., a first- or second-year course), the course prerequisites (i.e., completion of a clinical experience in mental health in a previous course), and knowledge of the program itself (i.e., traditional four-year or two-year accelerated baccalaureate degree) will provide the CI with important general information regarding the students' theoretical preparation and practical skills. Because of the trend in decreased opportunities for direct-care clinical placements in much of Canada, and certainly because of the COVID-19 pandemic that began in 2020, students who have no exposure to patient care activities may be less confident when compared to past students who had the advantage of such experiences. With a thorough understanding of the curriculum in which they teach, the CI can consider the assessment of individual student learning needs. Student needs assessment is covered in an earlier chapter in this textbook.

Although students have acquired nursing practice knowledge in the classroom and have met the clinical course outcomes in previous courses, each student may have had different clinical experiences. A student may not have been exposed to certain skills because the clinical opportunity was not available on the assigned unit, shift, or day, or because of the type of patient that they had been assigned. If a student had been placed at an agency before, the student may already have knowledge of the physical layout, infrastructure, or general policies and procedures of that agency. Based on these anticipated variations, the CI should assess learning needs early in the placement. With the often-limited time spent in clinical teaching, the sooner learning needs are identified, the sooner students can be supported in meeting course outcomes.

Planning for Successful Clinical Evaluation

As a result of the initial assessment by the CI and the students' own self-assessments, understanding of the course outcomes may be reinforced through the creation of personal learning plans for the clinical course experience at the start of the course (Calleja et al., 2016). Personal learning plans that are created by students with the input of a CI or preceptor must align with the course outcomes.

While a Canadian study emphasized that CIs may not necessarily have the skills to provide effective feedback to support students' self-regulated learning (Filice et al., 2020), formulation of a personal learning plan by each student facilitates CI-student collaboration in the overall clinical evaluation process, and the development of self-assessment skills, which is an important characteristic of a self-regulated professional. It is observed, however, that self-assessment as a primary source of evaluation is unreliable and inaccurate (Hadid, 2017). Therefore, course designers and CIs need to be cautious that a student's personal learning plan goals are not the sole focus of measurement for success in the course and that the approved course outcomes are achieved to support progress across the curriculum.

Personal goals are student-specific to support an area of interest and past clinical learning and need not reflect the whole of the course goals. A personal goal created by a student that relates to pediatric care for a clinical course on adult acute care is not appropriate, no matter the learning needs or gaps identified. Such personal learning plans can be adapted based on formative feedback and in response to the dynamic nature of the clinical setting (e.g., a student may plan to become more proficient at a specific task, but if the opportunity does not occur on the assigned unit, this may need to change).

The development of a learning plan to support the individual, initial assessment of a student's needs includes a goal written in the SMART format (specific, measurable, achievable, relevant/realistic, and time-bound); the course outcome or outcomes associated with the goal; the objectives or tasks that need to be accomplished to meet that goal; available resources; a deadline or target date; and the criteria for achievement (evidence of completion). See Figure 7.3 for a template for a student's personal learning plan.

Figure 7.3 *Personal Clinical Learning Plan*

Personal goal	Course outcome(s) associated with goal	Objectives to support personal goal	Resources to access	Target date	Evidence of achievement
1.		a. b.			
2.		...			
3.					
...					

The initial assessment of a student (or groups of students) sets the stage for teaching and establishing plans for achievement of clinical outcomes. This assessment is an important first step in a meaningful and clear clinical evaluation process. The general expectations and an understanding of what will be involved in this process lay the groundwork for ongoing, formative feedback that will provide students with guidance for improving their performance. In the next section, formative approaches are further discussed.

Formative Evaluation to Support Clinical Learning

Formative feedback and evaluation are critical to a student's development of new practice knowledge and skills, and to their progression in the program. Without regular and relevant input on performance, students may not improve or meet the course outcomes. The CI must therefore plan to employ various methods for gathering information on student performance, which form a basis for ongoing feedback.

Approaches for the Ongoing Collection of Data and Performance Analysis

Clinical evaluation strategies are employed within the course to establish whether students are achieving desired clinical outcomes. Building on the initial assessment of student knowledge and learning needs, a variety of approaches may be used to gather information about performance. These include planned activities such as direct observation and anecdotal notetaking by the CI, a review of student-completed checklists, and assessment of short clinical assignments or a student's clinical portfolio (Oermann et al., 2022). Other informal data may be obtained through reports from other health care professionals, peers, or patients interacting with the student. Each of these assessment strategies are discussed more fully below.

- *Direct observation and anecdotal notes.* In a survey of CIs in the United States and Canada, most respondents indicated that they use anecdotal notes for record-keeping (Hall, 2013). Anecdotal notes about students' performance are useful because with the passage of time, details about demonstrated practice may be difficult to recall. Whether these notes are handwritten or recorded electronically, notations should be shared often with the student to support ongoing feedback and formal evaluation (Quance, 2016).
- *Checklists.* As a quick way to record skills or behaviours, CIs and students can use these checklists to keep track of tasks that need to be completed over time or for noting specific steps that have been accomplished in a single activity.

- *Clinical assignments.* Written assignments may be used to gather information on students' problem-solving and clinical reasoning processes (Oermann & Gaberson, 2017); these may include reflective and self-assessment notes, care plans, concept maps, case studies, post-conference presentations, or portfolios (a collection of projects, materials and resources developed by the students during the clinical experience). Each assignment should be carefully designed with a specific purpose and defined expectations for how it will contribute to the student's learning experience.
- *Informal data from others.* A student's peers and health care professionals working with the student may provide input on performance. Verification or confirmation of such input is important so that a CI's decisions are not made based on a misunderstanding of what is seen on expectations that a student knows material that is beyond their level.

Any documentation needs to be kept confidential according to Canadian and provincial and territorial privacy legislation and institutional policy, as appropriate.

Selection of any of these approaches for collecting information related to student performance is based on the clinical environment, level of the student, the conventions of the academic institution, and the length of available time for the students to demonstrate outcomes. Virtual or screen-based learning may also be incorporated to augment clinical learning; such adjuncts would be included in the program or course delivery plan. Some of the additional data that are assessed may be incorporated into the grading structure. No matter the approach, the CI continues to verify the data collected on the students' performance by providing them with prompt feedback and with reference to the competency expectations of the clinical experience.

The CI always uses appropriate, inclusive, and professional language and avoids derogatory descriptions of a student's thinking or actions when speaking to students or in documenting any evaluation. Modelling respectful and collegial attitudes and behaviours of a registered nurse by the CI, for instance, during interactions with patients and the unit staff can also positively reinforce desired student performance. Conversely, poor, disrespectful behaviours and comments are likely to have the opposite effect. Various principles may be used by the CI to provide feedback in a meaningful way.

General Feedback Principles for Clinical Performance Evaluation

Chickering and Gamson (1987) identified principles of good practice when providing feedback to students; these are essential to establishing a positive learning environment. Particularly, the principles of communicating high expectations and giving prompt feedback support the clinical evaluation process and the progression of student learning.

Providing ongoing feedback throughout a students' clinical experience, based on the data collected, is necessary for several reasons. Students require input on their behaviours and skills to continually improve their performance and to correct any safety issues. Communicating with a student about their learning also helps them learn how to receive feedback in a professional manner and how to ask for clarification as needed. In addition, continual feedback can keep students focused on the clinical course outcomes. Feedback to students during the clinical evaluation process should be the following:

- *Constructive and relevant.* Providing constructive comments to students, with clear and accurate examples of behaviours, is necessary. These comments should relate to the clinical course outcomes and reflect the level of the student (e.g., beginning students may require more detail). Encouragement includes acknowledgement of positive achievements, allows room for error, and identifies an expectation for improvement. Student self-assessment can be sought first; feedback can be more meaningful if the student self-assesses first, uncovering what is relevant to them (Gigante et al., 2011).

- *Specific.* Individualized to a student's learning needs and with an understanding of their preferred learning style, feedback in the clinical evaluation process should be specific to each student.
- *Timely.* Conveying feedback to students about a particular incident needs to occur promptly. This means that when an action by a student is observed, or once the CI is aware, positive feedback or ways to improve should be shared as soon as is feasible. However, the CI needs to avoid correcting a mistake too quickly or telling the student what the next step is. A delay in sharing feedback prevents the student from addressing their own behaviours, reduces recall of the nuances of the issue for both the CI and the student, and renders the feedback less meaningful. Feedback is often associated with a deadline to improve.
- *Respectful.* Conversations with students about improvements to their personal performance should occur privately, and out of earshot of other students, patients, and agency staff. While a student may be observed making a mistake in the provision of direct care, gentle redirection or removal of the student from the situation can occur first, and then more detailed one-on-one feedback can immediately follow the experience to reinforce learning. Inclusive and fair approaches assist students to overcome feelings of anxiety, lack of confidence, or being overwhelmed, and respect and value students' work and efforts. Questions and comments should be reflective, supportive, and elicit student reflection, rather than being forceful, confrontational, and threatening. See Figure 7.4.

Figure 7.4 *Examples of Comments to Support Student Learning*

Less supportive comment	More supportive comment
"I need to speak with you about a problem you are having."	"I asked you to meet with me because I care about your success."
"You did [skill] without proper preparation and did not prioritize your actions."	"I just observed that you performed [skill] and noticed that you had some challenges; can you tell me about what happened?"
"Your care was unsafe, and the patient could have been harmed."	"If you were the patient and knew this happened, would you feel that you were receiving safe care?"
"If you continue this way, I am going to have to fail you."	"Let's work out a plan for you to improve and meet the course outcomes."

Source: Based on Altmiller (2016) and Oermann and Gaberson (2017).

Consistency in the application of general feedback principles can facilitate the clinical evaluation process, whether for in-person clinical experiences or for simulation or screen-based clinical adjunct activities.

Ongoing Feedback of the Student During a Clinical Course

Learning evolves over time; this is an expectation that is shared at the beginning of the clinical evaluation process, and is reinforced through ongoing, formative feedback provided to the student. With the information gained from observing and collecting data on a student's clinical performance, and a grounding in best practices for feedback, the CI can complete a formative evaluation. Ongoing, individualized feedback can be shared regularly and informally with the student, but typically, and often at the midpoint in the course, a more formal discussion is scheduled.

The purpose of the mid-course evaluation is to provide formative feedback on performance. It allows the CI and student to collaborate on what behaviours should continue to be reinforced, what to correct or improve on, and to ascertain or map the student's progress towards meeting the course outcomes. Collaboration is necessary to ensure that a CI's perceptions about a student's performance and thinking are interpreted correctly, and that the student is clear on how they are doing. Documentation of this formal discussion is part of the academic record. It is referred to at the end of the course to gauge improvement and to judge the student's overall development of the required knowledge and skills.

Remediation Planning to Support Progression

Clinical experiences can be anxiety-provoking; evaluation of clinical performance is a stressful occurrence for students. Early identification of a student who is having difficulties improving or demonstrating the required competencies is important to support the student and to mitigate escalation of anxiety (Houghton, 2016). Ongoing assessment of a student's activities contributes to accurate and timely communication of performance issues.

Relating to the principle of timely feedback, the earlier that challenges are noticed and communicated, the sooner that student can receive specific input on what they need to do to improve (Killam et al., 2011). Therefore, this aspect of the formative component of the clinical evaluation process is critical to a student's success in the course.

A learning contract, also known as a remediation or progression plan, is needed when the CI (or an assigned preceptor) identifies problems with a student's knowledge, behaviour, or clinical performance that may pose a barrier to the achievement of the required clinical course outcomes. To create a learning contract or remediation plan with an underperforming student, the CI or preceptor and student meet and discuss ways to address the identified gaps using the following steps (Meyer & Peters, 2010):

- General concerns and need for remediation are communicated promptly after an event or as indicated.
- The CI provides a written, non-judgemental, specific, concise, and factual description of the event(s), in relation to the course outcomes or expected competencies.
- The student provides written feedback on perceived learning needs in relation to the event.
- The CI and student meet to collaborate on options to address learning gaps.
- Together, the CI and student create a plan of action that includes specific, actionable activities and a target date.

Therefore, documenting such learning contracts or remediation plans with students who are having difficulty meeting the course outcomes or competencies include a summary of the student's and CI's perception of the performance issue, a detailed list of specific issues to address (listed separately), methods and resources to achieve improved performance, evidence of achievement, a deadline for completing the remediation activity, and any relevant notes about how that outcome can occur. This forms a contract for learning. A summary statement by the student and CI on the remediation is written at the completion of the plan. The signed plan remains part of the academic record (see Figure 7.5).

It should be communicated to the student that any learning contract or remediation plan is always included as a component of the clinical course requirements. Additionally, students need to be made aware that improvement in performance must be sustained at the required level, and that the completion of the remediation plan does not guarantee a passing grade in the clinical course as all the remaining requirements must also be fully met.

As with all CI-student interactions, a positive and respectful learning environment is maintained. Students feel vulnerable when progressing through a remediation plan, and so confidentiality, inclusiveness, transparency, and fairness are paramount. As discussed further in Chapter 6, good learning contracts or plans include links to professional standards and practice standards. Both students and CIs need to understand how learning plans support students in achieving the knowledge skills and attitudes expected by their profession. Similarly, clear communication of any related policies that apply to the remediation process, particularly if a mistake was made (such as a medication administration error), should occur. This includes clinical agency policy as it applies to students performing patient care and academic progression policies. Policies can be presented to students as a mechanism for guidance and for seeking solutions.

Figure 7.5 *Remediation Plan Example – Contract*

Course Information: Program/Year:						
Student self-assessment of clinical performance issue			CI observations of clinical performance issue:		
Clinical performance issue(s) to be addressed	Required activities to address issue	Resources (lab practice, simulation, etc.)	Evidence of achievement	Target date	Completion notes
1.					
2.					
…					
Student summary comments:			CI summary comments:		
Signatures: Date:						

Students who are not initially meeting the course outcomes, or who are underperforming, can be permitted to continue to participate in the clinical environment with the approval of the agency (if this is required). However, if a student has demonstrated unsafe performance, the risk of allowing them to continue in the health care setting may be deemed too high, and so removal from the clinical environment may be necessary. A remediation plan and the program's academic policies provide guidance in such cases. Remediation may therefore occur in the laboratory using simulation and other skill-building activities until the student can demonstrate safe practice and return to providing care for patients.

Summative Evaluation of Student Clinical Performance

While various approaches can be taken for establishing a collaborative relationship between the CI and student that supports students' learning and growth (refer to Chapter 3), the CI is ultimately responsible for making a judgement of the students' performance in the clinical setting. As the last component of the clinical evaluation process, the summative evaluation requires the CI to make a judgement that stands as the final grade for the clinical course.

Formulation of the final evaluation involves analysis of an individual student's performance across the course. Because students have had ongoing assessment and received formative feedback, the outcome of a student's final clinical course evaluation should not be a surprise to the student; it should be a summation of what has been shared to that point and the final judgement that has been documented.

The challenges for communicating clearly and meaningfully can be addressed by using a structured clinical evaluation tool that incorporates formative and summative evaluation of the student.

Formal Clinical Evaluation Tools

A formal tool for structuring the clinical evaluation process serves to guide the CI about what to observe during the clinical experience, and to frame feedback in an objective and specific manner, so that the student's achievement of the clinical course outcomes is documented. In some tools, requirements that are beyond, or in addition to, the course outcomes are also evaluated as ever-present professional behaviours. These include person-centred care, evidence-informed decision-making, interprofessional collaboration, and safety (Altmiller, 2019). An example of a comprehensive clinical evaluation tool is provided in Figure 7.6.

Figure 7.6 *Clinical Evaluation Tool Example*

Course Information:

Program/Year:

Course outcome	Associated clinical competencies (course, specialty, or regulatory, etc.)	Student self-reflection/ analysis	CI comments	Student self-reflection/ analysis	CI comments
		Formative evaluation (passing/failing; satisfactory, needs improvement)		Summative evaluation (pass/fail; satisfactory, unsatisfactory)	
1.					
2.					
...					

Final grade:

Signatures:

Date:

The students' personal learning activities (see Figure 7.3) can be referred to in the student's formative and summative self-reflection and analysis regarding how course outcomes and clinical competencies have been achieved. This self-examination, as a component of the formal clinical evaluation, reinforces professional requirements for reflection on practice and lifelong learning. When completed before the CI's comments are added, the student's self-evaluation can reveal their skills related to insight and planning for self-improvement.

Regular input on formal evaluation tools from the CI and students, as the end-users of the document, should be considered to ensure that the criteria and clinical outcomes remain relevant and applicable to the activities of students in the clinical setting. Students should have access to the tool at the outset of the course so they know the format for evaluating their performance. The tool can be reviewed annually and modified as required.

Grading

The grading conventions of academic institutions for a student's clinical performance are often a *pass-fail* rating or may include further gradations of a pass, such as *competent*, *satisfactory*, or *above expectations*. If such gradations or a letter grade are used, they are qualified by clear descriptions that align with *pass-fail* performance. Numeric grades are not typically assigned to clinical performance and may be difficult to justify (Oermann & Gaberson, 2017). Requirements either for meeting all outcomes in the course or for earning a passing grade in only key critical competencies should also be communicated as part of the grading approach. These expectations should be identified in the course syllabus or outline at the outset of the course.

Clinical evaluation may be norm-referenced or criterion-referenced and may be a combination of both. *Criterion-referenced* evaluation occurs when students' clinical performance is compared with predetermined standards and outcomes (McDonald, 2017), such as course goals or practicum competencies. Students are judged as either meeting the standard or not. *Norm-referenced* evaluation compares a student's performance with that of other students at the same level, based on a combination of assessment results (McDonald, 2017). In this circumstance, a student may be rated as *average* or *above average*. This requires that the CI understands what a student's standard performance in the course (or program) should look like.

Rating performance and assigning a grade to clinical practice is a challenge. A student who performs well and is evaluated based on a patient care experience that was predictable versus a student in the same group who performs less well but is evaluated on a patient care experience that was continually changing is a difficult comparison for a CI. Would the first student who performs well without a challenge have also performed well in that changing patient care experience? Is comparison reasonable?

Pass or fail grade categories may provide limited feedback to a student, and vague definitions of competencies may contribute to passing a failing student to give them the benefit of the doubt (Heaslip & Scammell, 2012). A review by Almalkawi et al. (2018) suggested that there is a need to distinguish between levels of competence and to establish clear communication of evaluation outcomes. Descriptors or scoring rubrics for defined performance levels are needed in feedback tools to support progress and to facilitate a final judgement and assignment of a grade. Behaviours that relate to safety, prompting, confidence, and use of theoretical knowledge may be referred to (Kopp, 2018). Possible options for creating levelled descriptors are offered in Table 2 and can be modified to reflect specific course requirements.

The Unsuccessful Student

Despite communication of clear outcomes, individualized teaching approaches, and a supportive learning environment, some students may not be able to achieve the outcomes to pass a clinical course. This experience can be devastating to the student and distressing to the CI.

Canadian data included in a 2020 study revealed that common issues in student failures in clinical performance were poor communication, inadequate knowledge and clinical incompetence, and unprofessional behaviours (Rojo et al., 2020). Other issues such as a lack of awareness and insight have also been noted in reviews by Canadian scholars (Killam et al., 2011; Scanlan & Chernomas, 2016). DeBrew and Lewallen (2014) noted that unsuccessful student behaviours include poor communication, failure to progress even after a supportive plan is created, and unsafe medication administration.

Figure 7.7 *Sample Descriptors for Levelled Student Clinical Performance*

Possible ratings	Descriptors
Satisfactory Pass	The student is performing *above the minimum competency level* that is appropriate for the course, in consideration of the practice environment, with some, or minimal assistance: • performs safely • applies theory and evidence most of the time • builds organizational skills and prioritization • demonstrates clinical reasoning and judgement skills • identifies situations where assistance is needed; seeks help • communicates patient situations or community needs accurately
Needs Improvement Passing	The student is performing *at the minimum competency level* that is appropriate for the course, in consideration of the practice environment, with regular assistance: • performs safely with direction • applies theory and evidence when prompted • inconsistently applies identified organizational skills and prioritization to care or course activities • demonstrates clinical reasoning and judgement skills when prompted • identifies situations where assistance is needed; inconsistently seeks appropriate help • communicates patient situations or community needs with minimal but key information
Unsatisfactory Failing Fail	The student is performing *below the minimum competency level* that is appropriate for the course, in consideration of the practice environment, requiring continual assistance and supervision: • performs unsafely • is unable to apply theory and evidence • is unable to organize or prioritize care or course activities • is unable to demonstrate clinical reasoning and judgement skills when prompted • does not identify situations where assistance is needed, and does not seek help • communicates patient situations or community needs inaccurately, missing key points

McGregor (2007), a Canadian nurse educator, examined student failures and discussed that the academic system needs to acknowledge and support students who are unsuccessful, that some students need more time and flexible options to be successful in clinical practice, and that more support, rather than a disconnect, is required for struggling students. Therefore, discussions with a student who is at risk of failing, or who has failed a clinical course component, should focus on their inability to demonstrate the course outcomes, rather than the personal perspectives of the CI, or the personal attributes of the student.

Instead of the CI following any desire to provide personal counselling to a student who has external issues that may be affecting their clinical performance, they should refer students to the appropriate counselling, social, or mental health services; while supportive, the CI needs to maintain a professional perspective to provide a fair evaluation. In addition, all policies relating to remediation planning and unsafe clinical performance or failure of a clinical course should be followed and made clear to the student. Advice from other academic faculty in administrative positions can assist the student to navigate these policies and provide a path to repeating the course and continuing in the program if that is an option. Fairness and transparency are key to student support.

Framing failure as a positive experience of growth can be difficult (Melrose et al., 2015). If the option for repeating the course is provided, looking at the experience as an opportunity to take more time to acquire the necessary knowledge and skill to learn can be useful to the student and the CI.

Implications of the Clinical Evaluation Process for the CI

A student's individual clinical performance evaluation is situated in the context of busy health care environments, is influenced by personal issues and group dynamics and relationships, and occurs in the public domain. These factors contribute to complexity of decision-making for the CI. The impact on the CI when engaged in decision-making about a failing student can be a lonely, emotional experience and may include feelings of inadequacy or failure in their own role (Larocque & Luhanga, 2013).

The concept of *failure to fail* is a documented phenomenon that has been present in the literature for decades (Lankshear, 1990; Rutkowski, 2007). Hughes et al. (2019) indicated that some CIs passed students who they felt were failing and that the CIs reported inadequate opportunities to fully assess students. Nugent and colleagues (2020) described that the most significant barrier to failing students was a lack of availability of supportive evidence to substantiate the failure, and that while CIs will recommend a failure to students that are performing below the requirements, there remains a reluctance to fail among some CIs or preceptors who need more support throughout the clinical evaluation process.

Communication between the CI and other faculty can provide opportunities for greater support for providing formative and summative evaluation of students. Orientation to the CI role and to the individual courses can also assist with familiarizing the CI with course requirements that students need to attain. Overall, the aim is to ensure that both the CI and students feel supported in the clinical evaluation process and, ultimately, to enable students to achieve success in the nursing program.

Summary

This chapter presented the complexities of evaluation in the clinical setting. Differentiation between assessment and evaluation, and formative and summative evaluation activities were defined and described in the context of measuring student performance.

The initial assessment of the student, understanding of student needs in relation to the course and the program, personal learning plans, and course outcomes as the foundation for clinical learning were discussed. The significance of formative feedback and how to deliver respectful and meaningful information to the student, as well as ways to create progression or remediation plans, were reviewed. Methods to evaluate clinical performance in addition to observation, such as written work and students' self-reflections, were covered.

Summative evaluations, compared to formative feedback, were described, as well as strategies related to communication and documentation of the acquisition of learning outcomes in relation to prescribed expectations. The summative evaluation of a student, whether they have performed well or poorly, needs to be constructive, clear, relevant, and related to the course outcomes and identified requirements. The challenges of struggling students were captured and recommendations for supporting both the student and the CI were outlined.

Conclusion

Clinical evaluation in Canada, aligning with the nursing education processes that are documented in the literature, is a critical process for facilitating the success of students in a nursing program and for supporting graduates as they enter nursing practice. Course outcomes and competencies for thinking and acting like a nurse are the foundation for how students are assessed and evaluated in nursing education. As health care environments become more challenging to teach and learn in, the CI needs to understand and appreciate the tentativeness and work in progress of the student in training—students have much to learn, gain confidence in, and master. The level of the program has an impact on expectations of either simple or complex application of knowledge and dependent or independent student performance for determining successful achievement of outcomes.

References

Almalkawi, I., Jester, R., & Terry, L. (2018). Exploring mentors' interpretation of terminology and levels of competence when assessing nursing students: An integrative review. *Nurse Education Today*, 69, 95. https://doi.org/10.1016/j.nedt.2018.07.003

Altmiller, G. (2016). Strategies for providing constructive feedback to students. *Nurse Educator*, 41(3), 118-119. https://doi.org/10.1097/NNE.0000000000000227

Altmiller, G. (2019). Content validation of quality and safety education for nurses prelicensure clinical evaluation tools. *Nurse Educator*, 44(3), 118-121. https://doi.org/10.1097/nne.0000000000000656

Baker, C. (2020). Clinical nursing education in the Canadian context. In K. Page-Cutrara & P. Bradley (Eds.), *The role of the nurse educator in Canada* (pp. 220-237). Canadian Association of Schools of Nursing.

Brookhart, S. M., & Nitko, A. J. (2015). *Educational assessment of students* (7th ed.). Pearson.

Calleja, P., Harvey, T., Fox, A., & Carmichael, M. (2016). Feedback and clinical practice improvement: A tool to assist workplace supervisors and students. *Nurse Education in Practice*, 17, 167-173. https://doi.org/10.1016/j.nepr.2015.11.009

Chickering, A., & Gamson, Z. (1987). Seven principles for good practice in undergraduate education. *American Association for Higher Education AAHE Bulletin*, 39(7), 3-7. https://doi.org/10.25071/1497-3170.2711

DeBrew, J. K., & Lewallen, L. P. (2014). To pass or to fail? understanding the factors considered by faculty in the clinical evaluation of nursing students. *Nurse Education Today*, 34(4), 631. https://doi.org/10.1016/j.nedt.2013.05.014

Fainstad, T. L., McClintock, A. H., & Yarris, L. M. (2021). Bias in assessment: name, reframe, and check in. *The Clinical Teacher*. https://doi.org/10.1111/tct.13351

Filice, S., Tregunno, D., Edge, D., & Egan, R. (2020). Re-imaging clinical education: The interdependence of the self-regulated clinical teacher and nursing student. *International Journal of Nursing Education Scholarship*, 17(1). https://doi.org/10.1515/ijnes-2019-0056

Gaba, D. (2004). The future vision of simulation in healthcare. *BMJ Quality & Safety*, 13 (Suppl. 1), i2-i10. http://doi.org/10.1136/qshc.2004.009878

Gigante, J., Dell, M., & Sharkey, A. (2011). Getting beyond "good job": How to give effective feedback. *Pediatrics*, 127, 205-207. https://doi.org/10.1542/peds.2010-3351

Hadid, S. (2017). Factors influencing nursing student self-assessment in relation to instructor assessment. *Journal of Nursing Education*, 56(2), 70-76. https://doi.org/10.3928/01484834-20170123-03

Hall, M. A. (2013). An expanded look at evaluating clinical performance: Faculty use of anecdotal notes in the U.S. and Canada. *Nurse Education in Practice*, 13(4), 271-276. https://doi.org/10.1016/j.nepr.2013.02.001

Heaslip, V., & Scammell, J. M. E. (2012). Failing underperforming students: The role of grading in practice assessment. *Nurse Education in Practice*, 12(2), 95-100. https://doi.org/10.1016/j.nepr.2011.08.003

Lankshear, A. (1990). Failure to fail: The teacher's dilemma. *Nursing Standard*, 4(20), 35-37.

Houghton, T. (2016). Assessment and accountability: Part 2 – managing failing students. *Nursing Standard*, 30(41), 41. https://doi.org/10.7748/ns.30.41.41.s44

Hughes, L. J., Mitchell, M. L., & Johnston, A. N. (2019). Just how bad does it have to be? industry and academic assessors' experiences of failing to fail – A descriptive study. *Nurse Education Today*, 76, 206. https://doi.org/10.1016/j.nedt.2019.02.011

Killam, L., Luhanga, F., & Bakker, D. (2011). Characteristics of unsafe undergraduate nursing students in clinical practice: An integrative literature review. *Journal of Nursing Education, 50*(8), 437–446. https://doi.org/10.3928/01484834-20110517-05

Kopp, M. L. (2018). A standardized clinical performance grading rubric: Reliability assessment. *Journal of Nursing Education, 57*(9), 544–548. https://doi.org/10.3928/01484834-20180815-06

Larocque, S., & Luhanga, F. L. (2013). Exploring the issue of failure to fail in a nursing program. *International Journal of Nursing Education Scholarship, 10*(1). https://doi.org/10.1515/ijnes-2012-0037

Leighton, K., Kardong-Edgren, K., McNelis, A., Foisy-Doll, C., & Sullo, E. (2021). Traditional clinical outcomes in prelicensure nursing education: An empty systematic review. *Journal of Nursing Education, 60*(3), 136–142. https://doi.org/10.3928/01484834-20210222-03

Lewallen, L. P., & Van Horn, E. R. (2019). The state of the science on clinical evaluation in nursing education. *Nursing Education Perspectives, 40*(1), 4–10. https://doi.org/10.1097/01.nep.0000000000000376

McDonald, M. (2017). *The nurse educator's guide to assessing learning outcomes*. Jones & Bartlett.

McGregor, A. (2007). Academic success, clinical failure: Struggling practices of a failing student. *Journal of Nursing Education, 46*(11), 504–511. https://doi.org/10.3928/01484834-20071101-05

Melrose, S., Park, C., & Perry, B. (2015). *Creative clinical teaching in the health professions*. AU Press. https://clinicalteaching.pressbooks.com

Meyer, B., & Peters, J. (2010). An understanding approach to managing student issues. *Nurse Educator, 35*(2), 54–55. https://doi.org/10.1097/NNE.0b013e3181ced869

Oermann, M. H., De Gagne, J. C., & Phillips, B. (2022). *Teaching in nursing and the role of the educator* (3rd ed.). Springer.

Nugent, O., Lydon, C., Part, S., Dennehy, C., Fenn, H., Keane, L., Prizeman, G., & Timmins, F. (2020). Who is failing who? A survey exploration of the barriers & enablers to accurate decision making when nursing students' competence is below required standards. *Nursing Education in Practice, 45*. https://doi.org/10.1016/j.nepr.2020.102791

Oermann, M. H., & Gaberson, K. B. (2017). *Evaluation and testing in nursing education* (5th ed.). Springer.

Quance, M. A. (2016). Nursing students' perceptions of anecdotal notes as formative feedback. *International Journal of Nursing Education Scholarship, 13*(1), 75–85. https://doi.org/10.1515/ijnes-2015-0053

Rojo, J., Ramjan, L. M., Hunt, L., & Salamonson, Y. (2020). Nursing students' clinical performance issues and the facilitator's perspective: A scoping review. *Nurse Education in Practice, 48*. 102890 https://doi.org/10.1016/j.nepr.2020.102890

Rutkowski, K. (2007). Failure to fail: Assessing nursing students' competence during practice placements. *Nursing Standard, 22*(13), 35–40.

Scanlan, J. M., & Chernomas, W. M. (2016). Failing clinical practice & the unsafe student: A new perspective. *International Journal of Nursing Education Scholarship, 13*(1), 109–116. https://doi.org/10.1515/ijnes-2016-0021

CHAPTER 8

Legal and Ethical Dimensions of Clinical Instructing

Kathleen Leslie, Catharine Schiller, & Melissa Raby

When providing care to clients, nurses are responsible for following ethical, regulatory, and legal standards that guide practice. These standards also apply when nurses are supervising students in clinical environments. This chapter introduces clinical instructors to the ethical and legal principles that guide the supervision of nursing students in clinical placements.

Chapter Objectives

After completing the chapter, the reader will be able to
- explain how standards of practice, codes of ethics, and scopes of practice apply to the supervision of nursing students
- describe the basic components of a negligence claim and how they may apply to clinical instructors
- explore the components of educational appeals processes for clinical placements and how to prepare if a student appeals a clinical evaluation
- apply knowledge about legal and ethical dimensions of clinical instructing to mitigate risks and improve client safety
- identify relevant regulatory, legal, and ethical resources to support clinical instructors

Introduction

Clinical instructors (CIs) have a crucial role in ensuring nursing students are adequately supported to provide safe and competent care to their clients. As part of this role, CIs are responsible for assessing the performance of their students, providing adequate supervision to confirm students maintain legal and ethical standards, and ensuring students understand the standards and scopes of nursing practice that apply to their client population. In complex clinical environments, client safety is paramount and adverse events can occur if nursing students are not provided with competent supervision. Understanding the relevant regulatory, legal, and institutional implications of supervising students can help CIs mitigate risks and support safe and competent nursing care for clients.

Background and History

Legal and regulatory issues are not usually familiar territory for most CIs. While instructors may have encountered ethical issues in clinical practice, or even some thorny legal questions such as family disputes about substitute decision-making powers, most CIs have not been part of a negligence claim or found themselves in a regulatory hearing about their nursing licence. If a CI has taught students for some time, it is quite likely that they have encountered at least one student who wants to appeal their clinical grade or challenge their treatment by the instructor during a clinical placement. Unfortunately, misconceptions abound about the nature of legal or regulatory proceedings that can arise out of a clinical placement, as well as the process that the instructor may encounter if a student appeals a course outcome. None of these areas have been static; the expectations and role of a CI have developed in the same way that the nursing role has changed and grown over time. This chapter is intended to provide some clarity for the CI about the regulatory, civil law, and educational institution processes they may encounter as they fulfil their important responsibilities as teachers in a clinical setting.

Regulatory Issues

Nursing Regulation in Canada

Nurses in Canada are regulated health professionals. Regulation falls under the jurisdiction of the provinces and territories, and thus there are differences in nursing regulation across the country. The provincial and territorial governments set out a framework for regulation through legislation, but most of the day-to-day processes and activities for administering that framework are delegated to professional regulatory bodies.

Regulated nurses are likely familiar, to an extent, with their own nursing regulatory body. Nursing regulators in Canada are often called regulatory colleges (e.g., the College of Nurses of Ontario [CNO], the Nova Scotia College of Nurses [NSCN]). These regulatory colleges have the mandate of protecting the public by ensuring nurses are competent to provide safe care to their clients. This is a separate mandate from the professional advocacy functions of nursing associations and the labour relations function of unions. A few provinces have regulatory bodies with a dual mandate, performing both public protection and professional advancement roles, though this is an increasingly uncommon model as more provinces move to separate these functions into independent bodies.

To protect the public, nursing regulators aim to promote good nursing practice, prevent poor nursing practice, and intervene when nursing practice is unacceptable (NCSN, 2020). Nursing regulators typically do this by establishing requirements for initial entry to practice, managing registration and licensure, articulating and promoting standards of nursing practice, assessing continuing competence, and enforcing acceptable conduct through complaints and discipline processes (CNO, 2020a).

Standards of Practice

As part of their public protection role, nursing regulators in Canada establish, maintain, and enforce standards of practice for their nurse registrants/members. Generally, these standards of practice are authoritative statements that inform nurses of their accountabilities and let the public know what to expect of nurses (CNO, 2019b). Regulators also usually provide further practice guidelines or directions to help nurses understand and apply their practice expectations and obligations. Standards of practice, established by a nursing regulatory body, provide a benchmark for understanding reasonable and prudent nursing practice (College of Registered Nurses of Manitoba,

2018). Specific accountabilities for nursing educators may also be provided: for example, the CNO (2018) in its professional practice standard delineates specific indicators that nurses in educator roles can apply to ensure they are demonstrating these standards in practice. All CIs, as regulated nurses, are expected to be aware of and abide by the relevant standards of practice and other regulatory requirements for nursing practice in their jurisdiction.

Codes of Ethics

All regulated nurses follow a code of ethics. Ethical frameworks for nursing care, and relevant practice guidelines, are described by each nursing regulatory body. Some nursing regulators have adopted codes of ethics developed nationally (e.g., the *Code of Ethics for Registered Nurses* developed by the Canadian Nurses Association or the *Code of Ethics for Licensed Practical Nurses* developed by the Canadian Council of Practical Nurse Regulators) while some have developed an ethics standard to guide practice (e.g., the *Ethics Practice Standard* from the CNO or the *Ethical Practice Professional Standard* from the British Columbia College of Nurses and Midwives [BCCNM]). It is important that CIs model the integration of ethical principles into practice for students, provide guidance to students regarding ethical standards, and help students recognize and resolve ethical issues in practice. It is also important that CIs understand how ethical principles apply to their educational role, including maintaining professional relationships with students, ensuring clients understand and consent to students' involvement in their care, and assuring privacy and confidentiality of personal health information. See Box 8.1 for case examples.

Box 8.1 Case Examples

> A 2020 discipline decision at the CNO demonstrates what might happen when a CI engages in inappropriate behaviour with nursing students. In this case, the CI was found to have breached the standards of practice and committed professional misconduct after he engaged in a pattern of sexual behaviour towards two nursing students (CNO, 2020b). This behaviour included jokes of a sexual nature, staring at the students in an uncomfortable manner, winking at a student and rubbing her back, and sending an inappropriate voicemail to the effect of "I miss you. My wife is away." The discipline committee noted "aggravating factors" in the penalty, indicating that the CI had a supervisor role over nursing students, that "an important aspect of this role is to model appropriate professional behaviour," and that the CI took advantage of being in a position of power over these nursing students. The penalty in this case included a five-month suspension, an oral reprimand, mandated meetings with a regulatory expert, and mandatory employer notification for 18 months (CNO, 2019a).
>
> A 2016 discipline decision at the CNO also demonstrates the importance of respecting the privacy of personal health information of nursing students. In this case, the CI accessed the information of a nursing student in her clinical group after that nursing student had visited the emergency department where the CI worked and then disclosed this information to other nursing students in the clinical group. The CI was found to have committed professional misconduct. This case involved other instances of professional misconduct regarding inappropriate documentation, boundary violations, and privacy breaches, and the penalty included a four-month suspension, an oral reprimand, mandated meetings with a nursing expert, and mandatory employer notification for 18 months (CNO, 2016).

Scope of Practice

Scope of practice refers to activities that nurses are authorized, educated, and competent to perform (College & Association of Registered Nurses of Alberta, 2021). These activities are established through a definition of nursing practice provided in legislation and complemented by standards of practice established by nursing regulators (BCCNM, 2021). The actual scope of practice of each nurse requires practising within the overall legislative boundaries for scope of practice, but with specific actions determined by the needs of the client population, and limited by the nurse's individual competencies and relevant institutional policies (Schiller, 2015). Accordingly, scope of practice is a multi-layered and intricate relationship between the context of practice, individual nursing competencies, standards of practice, and specific jurisdictional legislation or regulation (Miller, 2020).

Practising within scope is an important aspect of providing safe and competent nursing care. CIs should ensure they are providing adequate supervision and guidance to students regarding scope of practice. CIs should be aware of any legislation or regulatory documents, as well as any institutional policies or guidelines, about the scope of practice for nursing students. In Ontario, for example, there is an exception authorizing performance of controlled acts (e.g., administering a medication by injection) under the *Regulated Health Professions Act* when that person is fulfilling requirements to become a member of a regulated health profession, the act is within the scope of practice of the profession, and the act is done under the supervision or direction of a member of the profession (e.g., the CI). In British Columbia, the nursing regulator states that nurses providing regulatory supervision of students may only authorize activities for which the student has gained competence through their education program, that are within the supervising nurse's scope of practice, and that are within the supervising nurse's individual competence (BCCNM, 2020). Nursing students in British Columbia are not authorized to perform any activity that affects client care unless these three conditions are met, and the activity is then authorized by a registrant of the BCCNM (BCCNM, 2020).

Regulatory Guidance for Supervision of Students

Supporting nursing students in practice is a professional responsibility for all regulated nurses, regardless of role. As the CNO (2021) states, all nurses are expected to act as mentors and are accountable to provide direction and share knowledge with new nurses or nursing students. CIs act in a formal support role and are expected to facilitate a learning environment that supports high quality patient care and professional growth for the students (CNO, 2021).

In British Columbia, the BCCNM provides a practice standard called regulatory supervision that sets out the requirements for nurses providing supervision to students or employed student registrants in practice. The BCCNM further details the process of supervising students as follows: understand the student's competence, authorize client care activities depending on this competence, set conditions for the activity (e.g., the CI being physically present), and manage risks to the clients to help ensure safe care (BCCNM, n.d.).

How does a regulator respond when nursing students make errors while they are completing a supervised clinical placement? According to the CNO (2018):

When a learner makes an error, examining the error's context is important. Nurses are not accountable for decisions or actions of other care providers when those actions were unknown and unforeseen. As such, a nurse is not accountable for the student's actions if their accountabilities to ensure safe patient care were met and if the nurse had no way of knowing the error was going to occur.

In British Columbia, the BCCNM states that nurses are accountable for decisions associated with regulatory supervision, including decisions made by the nursing student (BCCNM, 2020). Like the CNO, the BCCNM adds that nurses supervising students are not responsible or accountable for situations that could not be reasonably foreseen (BCCNM, 2020).

Clear and consistent communication from CIs, and an unfailing focus on client safety, can help mitigate risks of student errors in clinical placements. However, if a CI practices according to these established standards and appropriately assigns tasks to students, with proper training and oversight, and a nursing student still engages in inappropriate actions or makes an error, the CI is unlikely to be held accountable for the student's conduct.

Complaints and Discipline

It is natural to have some trepidation about the complaints and discipline process. However, this aspect of regulation is important for all nurses to understand, as it is one of the ways that nursing regulators work to ensure competent and safe nursing care for clients.

In fulfilling the mandate to protect the public, nursing regulators in each Canadian jurisdiction are typically required by the legislative framework to have a process for investigating complaints, conducting disciplinary hearings, and issuing sanctions to nurses who have committed professional misconduct or who have provided incompetent care (Hardcastle, 2019). This process is most often initiated by a complaint from a patient or family member. The process may also be initiated after a regulator receives a report about specific conduct or concerns from employers or colleagues. Sometimes these reports are mandatory, and it is important for nurses to know their obligations to report concerns about fellow health professionals to their regulatory body.

While there are differences across jurisdictions, the process for managing complaints or concerns about a nurse's practice typically involves reviewing the complaint first to determine if further action is required, then proceeding to an investigation if the complaint cannot be informally resolved and may have merit, and finally proceeding to a full discipline hearing if the investigation warrants. Discipline hearings are court-like processes. If the panel conducting the discipline hearing finds that there has been professional misconduct or incompetence, the panel will impose a sanction such as giving a reprimand, placing a limit or condition on the nurse's practice, or —in the most serious cases—revoking a nurse's licence to practice.

By following the appropriate standards and guidelines and properly supervising students, CIs reduce the risk that there will be a complaint about their care made to the nursing regulator. It is, however, still possible. If nurses receive a notice of a complaint about their nursing care from a regulatory body, legal assistance may be available through the Canadian Nurses Protective Society (CNPS), unions, or employers. There are also insurance options that nurses can purchase to provide legal assistance if they are responding to a complaint (e.g., the Supplementary Protection Program of the Canadian Nurses Protection Society or the Legal Assistance Program of the Registered Nurses' Association of Ontario). CIs who want to know about or discuss these options should contact their union, association, or the CNPS for more information.

Civil Issues

Civil Law Actions in Canada

There are two main types of legal cases in Canada's legal system: criminal and civil. Criminal law deals with violations of Canada's *Criminal Code* or other federal statutes. A crime is considered an offence against society. While it is possible for nurses to face criminal charges for offences such as diverting controlled substances or abusing clients, criminal conduct associated with nursing practice is – thankfully – rare. In this chapter, we focus on civil actions, where one party sues another to resolve a dispute or be compensated for a harm or loss. When an adverse event occurs while someone is receiving health care, serious harm can result. Sometimes the person who was harmed will seek compensation through a civil action claiming negligence.

Negligence

Negligence refers to careless or unreasonable conduct that causes harm or loss (Nelson & Ogbogu, 2018). In nursing, negligence can occur when a client is harmed as a result of a nurse's failure to do what a reasonable nurse would do in the same situation. The law of negligence is complex and nuanced. In this chapter, we provide a basic introduction to negligence and discuss how it may apply to CIs.

Patients have the right to expect competent nursing care even if that care is being provided by nursing students. If a patient receives an injury because of care provided by a nursing student, the patient may decide to sue for compensation. The patient may name multiple parties in their lawsuit, such as the nursing student, the CI, the school of nursing, and the clinical agency. Student nurses may be held personally liable for their own negligent acts and the CI may be held liable for negligence in supervision. For example, a patient may sue a CI if the patient believes that the CI failed to supervise the nursing student appropriately or assigned the student a task that the CI knew, or ought to have known, the nursing student was not competent to perform, and the patient suffered an injury or loss as a result.

To be successful in a negligence claim, four elements must be proved by the plaintiff (the party bringing the negligence action to court):

- A duty of care was owed to the plaintiff by the defendant.
- The defendant failed to meet the standard of care.
- The plaintiff suffered a harm.
- The defendant's failure to meet the standard of care was the cause of that harm.

Every case is based on the individual circumstances of that case, and liability must be proven on a balance of probabilities.

We will demonstrate these four elements as they would relate to a potential claim against a CI for harm caused by a student the instructor was supervising.

Element 1: Duty of care

In most negligence claims against health professionals, establishing a duty of care is not contentious. The relationship between health professionals and patients is sufficiently close and it is foreseeable that if the health professional fails to take reasonable care to protect the patient, the patient may suffer harm as a result. This is generally true of CIs as well and would likely not be at issue in most cases.

Element 2: Failure to meet the standard of care

Once a duty of care has been established, the next, and more contentious, step in proving negligence is showing there was a breach in the standard of care. Establishing the standard of care in a medical negligence case requires that the court determine what a reasonably competent health professional would have done in the circumstances that led to the patient's injury. If a patient alleged that a CI was negligent, the court would need to determine what a reasonably competent CI would have done while supervising nursing students in similar circumstances. The standards of practice and other regulatory documents (discussed above under Regulatory Issues), as well as previous court cases and expert witnesses, may be used to provide a benchmark for the standard of care.

Elements 3 and 4: Harm and causation

Finally, the plaintiff will need to show that harm was suffered because of the CI's breach of the standard of care. Most medical negligence claims involve physical injuries, though claims for foreseeable psychiatric injuries are also possible (Hardcastle, 2019). In a claim against a CI, a patient would need to prove that they would not have suffered the injury if the CI had met the standard of care by providing appropriate supervision of the nursing student. See Box 8.2 for a case example.

Box 8.2 *Case Example*

> In *Granger (Litigation Guardian of) v. Ottawa General Hospital*, a baby suffered severe brain damage after being deprived of oxygen during birth. The staff nurse caring for the mother was inexperienced and did not report that the fetal heart monitor showed a constant deceleration of the baby's heart rate. In this case, the nursing team leader was found negligent for failing to assign the novice staff nurse's duties appropriately and failing to supervise the novice nurse according to the appropriate standard of nursing care.

Overall, while it is possible for a CI to be held liable for harms caused to a patient because of a student's actions (or omissions), it would be difficult for a court to find negligence in the actions of a CI who was following the appropriate standards and guidelines and properly supervising students.

Mitigating Risks

By understanding your responsibilities and accountabilities, following the appropriate standards and guidelines, and providing adequate supervision to nursing students, you are unlikely to face a professional misconduct complaint or negligence claim. However, it is important to recognize and actively seek to mitigate risks as much as is reasonably possible to help ensure safe and competent client care while contributing positively to your students' clinical education.

Here are some further actions you can take that may help mitigate risks of clinical placements:
- Ensure students are properly oriented to the clinical area and discuss potential occupational safety issues (e.g., infection control, needlesticks, patient transfers) that students may not be aware of because of their inexperience (Patton & Lewallen, 2015).
- Plan ways to evaluate student competencies prior to assigning tasks and throughout the placement.
- Discuss and document safety incidents or concerns about student performance immediately and according to educational institution and clinical agency processes.

Professional liability protection is meant to ensure financial compensation is available for patients who have been harmed because of the nurse's negligence and to protect nurses from the financial consequences of a civil law claim (CNPS, 2019). Carrying a form of this insurance is a requirement for most regulated nurses in Canada. CIs should be aware of the requirements for professional liability protection that their nursing regulatory body has set and ensure they consistently maintain this insurance coverage.

Educational Institution Issues

It is almost inevitable that, at some point in their teaching career, a CI will encounter a student who is unable to meet the clinical course requirements and therefore cannot be given a passing grade. The regulatory and civil law processes described above are typically initiated by the patient (or the patient's family) and tend to unfold quite some time after any event of concern. However, educational institution processes arising out of an unsuccessful student clinical placement are almost invariably initiated by the student and will engage the instructor during or very soon after the term of interest. It is critical that CIs understand the expectations of their educational institutions related to student performance and the school processes that will be engaged in if a student appeals an unsuccessful course outcome.

There are multiple routes of appeal at an educational institution depending upon the nature of the issue; for example, non-academic misconduct (such as threats against a faculty member or fellow student), academic misconduct (such as plagiarism), grade appeals, and program removal or requirement to withdraw appeals. This section of the chapter will focus on grade appeals, although it is strongly recommended that CIs familiarize themselves with their institution's policies and procedures related to all of these appeal routes.

Before the Term Begins

Well before the school term begins, CIs will already be busy preparing their courses and trying to anticipate issues so that everything will run smoothly once students arrive. At least, that's the plan! It would be wonderful if every potential problem scenario could be anticipated and prevented by this behind-the-scenes hard work of CIs. However, we know that this will usually be an unrealistic expectation – there will be relatively few teaching experiences in which you will have foreseen all possible clinical scenarios, student challenges, and clinical group needs. What you *can* do however, is set yourself and your students up for the best possible chance for success by sharing clear expectations and having a solid understanding of what your school requires.

Course Syllabus

The course syllabus serves as the student's first impression of the course they are embarking upon, but also acts as an ongoing reference source for both student and teacher. To be considered fair, a syllabus must be sufficiently detailed so that course expectations are clearly delineated, and students can identify the standards they must meet to demonstrate learning and pass the course. The time invested by a teacher in fine-tuning this document will be repaid tenfold as everyone will be able to clearly see the roadmap the course is to follow and know what must be accomplished to successfully reach the end of that journey. At minimum, the syllabus should set out a description of the course, course goals/objectives, contact information for the instructor, the course schedule, the evaluative measures (assignments) that will be required and the grade weighting of each, expectations specific to the course (such as penalties for late submissions and assignment extension requests), and a reference to key educational institution policies and procedures of which students should be aware (such as those related to plagiarism). If a student appeals an unsuccessful grade in the course, the syllabus will be the first document any appeals committee will consider in determining if procedural fairness issues hampered student achievement.

Familiarizing Yourself with Policies and Procedures

As a clinician, you are already aware of the importance of becoming familiar with the unit- and agency-specific policies and procedures (P&P) of your health care facility. A school is no different; there may be P&P that are specific to your nursing department, as well as P&P related to your educational institution more broadly. Before the term begins, it is good practice for a CI to review key P&P at their educational institution. For example, an appeals process can follow a slightly different format at each school and the expectations of an instructor at each step in that process might also look slightly different. It will be well worth your time to review these P&P before the term begins to ensure that you understand the role you will be expected to play should such circumstances arise. For most educational institutions, these P&P will be available online and can easily be accessed by instructors.

Dealing with Student Performance Concerns

As you already know, it is best to deal with any student performance concerns at the time they occur in the clinical placement. Addressing subpar or problematic clinical performance right away gives students the best possible chance to truly understand the issue, apply constructive feedback to their practice, and demonstrate their learning. Unfortunately, what many CIs do *not* do consistently is create an accompanying documentation trail to demonstrate that concerns were actually raised with the student. Of course, not every learning discussion that occurs between student and teacher needs to be documented; in fact, a typical clinical shift will ideally result in many such discussions with each student – it is how knowledge is transferred and learning occurs. However, if a significant issue has arisen, or if a pattern of problematic practice has begun to show, it will always be best to start the documentation process sooner rather than later. It is also critical that such documentation be shared with the student rather than simply filed away by the teacher. Should the student later appeal an unsuccessful course outcome, and express concern that they were not given adequate notice of an issue or sufficient opportunities to correct their practice, an appeals committee will expect to see evidence of these discussions and communications between instructor and student. The importance of complete and ongoing communication about a recurring issue cannot be overstated when an instructor is asked to support the decision to issue a failing grade. If such a grade was issued because of a single but highly significant practice issue (rather than repeated problematic practices), an appeals committee will still want to know that the reason the student was deemed unsuccessful was communicated to them clearly, that the consequence was made explicit, and that the course failure was commensurate with the practice concern.

Learning Contracts

One way of demonstrating that clinical practice concerns were brought to the attention of a student is a learning contract. As explained in Chapter 6, a learning contract may also be known as a remediation or progression plan, depending upon the institution. This document has developed a bad reputation with many students and teachers and is often seen (or wielded) as a highly punitive teaching tool. However, the potential for learning contracts to yield very positive outcomes for both student and teacher is high. If a CI begins the placement with a group discussion about learning contracts, and their intentions with respect to using them, at least some of that student fear can be eased. A learning contract or remediation plan is simply a document that sets out expectations and priorities, for both students *and* their teachers, for their time together during that term so that everyone involved is clear about them. A good learning contract will explicitly link these expectations and priorities with professional standards and practice standards, so that everyone involved understands their importance and the reason why our profession will anticipate that its members can meet these expectations. A template for a student's learning contract or plan is presented in Chapter 6.

A learning contract should also set out any verbal or written communications that have already taken place about these expectations and, if appropriate, state a timeframe by which successful demonstration of the skill or outcome is expected. What the student needs to actually *do* to demonstrate change, and how they can expect the instructor to help them achieve that change (e.g., giving feedback on a reflective journal entry about the issue within a certain period of time so the student can apply that feedback with their next patient, or organizing another learning opportunity during the placement to demonstrate improved skills), should also be clearly stated in the document. The student should not walk away from reading a learning contract with a lack of clarity about what they need to do to be successful or what they can expect from their instructor as support in reaching that goal. Finally, a student should know from reading the document what the likely consequence will be if they do not meet the learning goals within the stated timeframe. Students often catastrophize the likely response of instructors to concerns in the student's clinical practice and anticipate that even a small issue will lead to their ejection from the unit and a failing course grade. Such emotional responses can be lightened by CI transparency and an explicit discussion of the linkages the teacher intends to draw between the area of concern and the consequences being considered (Schiller, 2020).

A Student Appeal

While many CIs are concerned about the possibility that a student might appeal an unsuccessful outcome, it is often the lack of familiarity with an appeal process that causes the most worry (Schiller, 2020). An academic appeal is a process of the educational institution in which a school's representative is asked to review a decision related to a student's academic progress. An appeal will not be decided in favour of the student simply because the student has expressed dissatisfaction with the teacher or their grade. At most schools, a student will have to be able to demonstrate that there are actually grounds for appeal:

- The CI reached the grade decision in some procedurally unfair way (such as failing to mark an assignment in accordance with the rubric or with the requirements stated in the course syllabus).
- The grade was reached by the CI on some basis other than academic achievement (such as bias or a conflict of interest).
- There were extenuating circumstances (such as bereavement or a major illness) that were outside of the student's control, that significantly impacted the student's academic performance, and that the CI did not appropriately consider when grading the student or deciding upon assignment-related requests such as due date extensions.

When considering an appeals process, it is common to think about the college or university Appeals Committee. However, that usually represents the final step in the process. *It is important to remember that the steps may vary between institutions*, but generally a student will need to formally request reconsideration of their course outcome in the following order:

1. Ask the CI to reconsider the grade that was imposed. Usually this involves a meeting or discussion between the instructor and the student where the student outlines the basis on which they are challenging the grade and the instructor either rejects the student's appeal or supports it.
2. If the instructor rejects the student's appeal, then the student can request that the head of the school's nursing department (such as a chair or a coordinator) consider if there are grounds for an appeal. That individual will collect/review information about the course and the student's grade from both the instructor and the student before issuing their decision in writing.
3. If the head of the nursing department rejects the student's appeal, then the student can request that the Dean responsible for the nursing department consider if there are grounds for an appeal. That individual will also collect/review information about the course and the student's grade before issuing their decision in writing.
4. If the Dean rejects the student's appeal, then the student can apply to the educational institution Appeals Committee and ask them to consider whether there are grounds for an appeal.

CI involvement with the steps involving the head of the nursing department and the Dean will usually look quite similar. Instructors will be asked to submit documents to help a decision-maker reach a conclusion about whether there are grounds for appeal; for example, an instructor may need to submit the course syllabus, student evaluations issued during the course, relevant communications between the student and the instructor, marked assignments, relevant student feedback provided by unit staff during the clinical placement, and any other documents that can shed light on the instructor's decision-making about this student (a clear, concise summary document outlining the key aspects of the situation can also be very helpful for decision makers). Instructors may also be asked to meet in-person or participate in a teleconference with any of the above-noted individuals to provide details or clarifications. This is one time when keeping detailed notes throughout the term can greatly assist an instructor in recalling the factors that resulted in key decisions and demonstrating that the student received key communications and feedback from the instructor in a timely fashion. It is also a time when a detailed learning contract that set out areas for improvement, expectations of the student and the instructor, timeframes in which change needed to be demonstrated, the format those changes were to take, and the consequences that would attach to inadequate improvement can be invaluable in supporting the instructor's assertions during an appeal.

The Appeals Committee of the Educational Institution

The Appeals Committee of an educational institution is a standing committee. It usually comprises faculty members from across the institution, as well as having undergraduate and/or graduate student representation. The appeals process is not technically a legal process in the sense that it does not follow court rules of evidence or procedure. However, it is a well-established expectation that any appeals process and decision-making will follow the "principles of natural justice," a legal and ethical concept aimed at ensuring that a process is fair and is seen to be fair (e.g., see *Harelkin v. University of Regina*; *Yao v. University of Saskatchewan*). The principles of natural justice include such requirements as the following:

- ensuring that those involved in the appeal receive adequate notice of the proceedings
- ensuring that all parties in the appeal are made aware of evidence that will be considered in decision-making
- ensuring that all parties in the appeal are given a chance to make their arguments and provide supporting documentation
- ensuring that no voting member of the Appeals Committee has been involved in a decision-making process related to the matter under appeal or has a reasonable apprehension of bias/conflict of interest (British Columbia Ombudsperson, 2018; Chewter, 1994; Forrest & Miller, 2008; Huscroft, 2012)

Once an appeal reaches the level of the educational institution Appeals Committee, there will likely be nothing more for the instructor to add to the written package that they submitted at an earlier step of the process. The Appeals Committee will ensure that the student has received a complete copy of that written package. The student will need to specify to the Appeals Committee, in writing, what they are appealing, the grounds for their appeal, and the requested remedy in the situation. The potential remedies that the Appeals Committee has the power to impose will be set out in the P&P of the educational institution.

CIs often wonder if a student will be permitted to have a lawyer represent them during the hearing. That depends on the P&P of the particular educational institution. Some schools do allow students to be represented by legal counsel and for that counsel to present the student's case/ask questions, or they may restrict the role of the lawyer to aiding the student but not acting as their advocate. Other schools allow the student to have a support person present, such as a family member or friend, who can be there to provide emotional support to the student but not substantively contribute to the process. Still other schools have mandated that the student cannot have anyone accompanying them during a hearing.

Before the hearing, voting members of the Appeals Committee will have received a comprehensive documentation package to review. This will contain all written information submitted by the student to support their appeal, as well as the written information submitted by the school (including documents prepared by the CI) to outline the appeal process to date and the reasons why the appeal has been rejected at previous steps of that process.

The process at the Appeals Committee hearing usually unfolds in a fairly standard manner. Introductions of all parties will occur, including the members of the Appeals Committee. The committee chair will then ask the student to outline the basis for their appeal. The CI will then be asked to explain their decision related to the student's grade or course outcome. The head of the department and the dean will then be asked if they have any other information to add to what is already stated in the documentation package. The committee members may ask clarifying questions of speakers at any point in the process. Finally, the student and the instructor are given an opportunity to make final comments to the committee before they deliberate. Because the hearing is not a legal process, there should not be "cross-examinations" of speakers although the chair may permit clarifying questions to be asked by the parties. After the hearing is complete, the Appeals Committee deliberates in-camera and then the committee chair issues a written decision to the student and the nursing department (typically with a copy to the CI as well).

The decision of the educational institution Appeals Committee is a final one, and there are usually no other routes of appeal within the institution. This is also typically reinforced within a school's appeals process P&P. See Box 8.3 for a case study.

Box 8.3 *Case Study*

> Rick is a novice CI, midway through supervising third year BScN students in their acute care rotation. One of Rick's students, Alejandra, has arrived to clinical more than 20 minutes late twice in recent weeks. Each time, she has been unaware of her patient assignment and is ill-prepared regarding prescribed medications and the daily care plans. After consulting with the course coordinator and reviewing the learning outcomes described in the course syllabus, Rick schedules a meeting with Alejandra to discuss her progress in the course.
>
> During their meeting, Rick and Alejandra review the course learning outcomes and, using specific examples, Rick informs Alejandra that she is currently not meeting the course objective of "Professional behaviour: Learner is accountable to providing quality patient care by consistently being prepared for the clinical day." Rick clearly states that Alejandra is at risk of failing the course and suggests that a learning contract be developed to facilitate her success. Alejandra states her understanding and agreement, and a learning contract is developed and implemented.
>
> In the following weeks, Rick notes that Alejandra arrives to clinical on time and is well-prepared for the day. In the remaining weeks of clinical, Rick focuses much of his attention on another student who struggles with time management. In the final two weeks of placement, Alejandra once again comes late to clinical and is not prepared for the day. When Rick writes Alejandra's final evaluation, he assigns her a failing grade as she has not consistently met the course objective discussed in the learning contract.
>
> To his surprise, Rick learns that Alejandra has filed a course appeal. Rick speaks with the course coordinator, reviews his documentation of Alejandra's behaviour, and informs the appeals committee that he stands by his decision to assign her a failing grade. Rick is informed that the appeal will be assessed by the Appeals Hearing Committee. Despite the immense stress associated with preparing for the hearing, Rick feels confident that his thorough documentation of Alejandra's behaviour will support his decision.

Upon conclusion of the hearing, Rick is informed that the course failure grade will not be upheld, and Alejandra will be given additional clinical time (supervised by another CI) to demonstrate her ability to meet the course objective in question. The Appeals Hearing Committee informs Rick that there were procedural errors with the way the learning contract was implemented; specifically, it was not revisited and reviewed after its initial creation, meaning Alejandra had assumed that she was successfully meeting the course outcomes. A lesson learned for Rick!

Summary

CIs are responsible for following ethical, regulatory, and legal standards that guide nursing practice and their supervision of nursing students in clinical placements. In this chapter, we introduced CIs to ethical and legal principles to help guide their important work in supervising students in clinical placements. We described how standards of practice, codes of ethics, and scopes of practice apply to the supervision of students; introduced CIs to the components of a medical negligence claim; and explained the policies and processes for managing student performance concerns that become subject to an institutional appeal. This knowledge can help CIs mitigate risks in supervising students and help improve patient safety.

Conclusion

Supervised clinical experiences are essential components of basic nursing education. CIs play a vital part in educating the next generation of nurses by sharing their knowledge, skills, and experiences in this challenging and important role. Mitigating risks to ensure a safe and ethical clinical experience for everyone involved, including patients, is a shared responsibility between institutions, instructors, the clinical facility, and students. Understanding the relevant regulatory, legal, and institutional implications of supervising nursing students is an important part of a CI's role.

Note: The information in this chapter provides an overview of potential legal and ethical issues in providing clinical education to nursing students in Canada. None of the information in this chapter is meant to provide legal advice. CIs should consult their regulatory body, educational institutions, clinical agencies, the CNPS, and/or legal counsel regarding specific questions or concerns.

References

British Columbia College of Nurses and Midwives. (n.d.). *Regulatory supervision*. https://www.bccnm.ca/RN/learning/regulatorysupervision/Pages/Default.aspx

British Columbia College of Nurses and Midwives. (2020). *Practice standard: Regulatory supervision of students*. https://www.bccnm.ca/RN/PracticeStandards/Pages/regulatorysupervision.aspx

British Columbia College of Nurses and Midwives. (2021). *Scope of practice: Standards, limits, conditions*. https://www.bccnm.ca/Documents/standards_practice/rn/RN_ScopeofPractice.pdf

British Columbia Ombudsperson. (2018). *Fairness in practice*. https://bcombudsperson.ca/guide/fairness-in-practice/

Canadian Nurses Protective Society. (2019). *Ask a lawyer: Employer-provided professional liability protection*. https://cnps.ca/article/ask-a-lawyer-employer-provided-professional-liability-protection/

Chewter, C. (1994). Justice in the university: Legal avenues for students. *Dalhousie Journal of Legal Studies*, 3(5), 105–136. https://digitalcommons.schulichlaw.dal.ca/djls

College & Association of Registered Nurses of Alberta. (2021). *Scope of practice for registered nurses*. https://nurses.ab.ca

College of Nurses of Ontario. (2016). *Discipline committee of the college of nurses of Ontario*. https://registry.cno.org/Search/OpenPublicRegisterDocument?PubliceRegisterDocumentId=bf545ec5-3332-ea11-940f-00155d3afcff

College of Nurses of Ontario. (2018). Professional standards, revised 2002. https://www.cno.org/globalassets/docs/prac/41006_profstds.pdf

College of Nurses of Ontario. (2019a). *Discipline committee of the college of nurses of Ontario*. https://www.cno.org/globalassets/2howweprotectthepublic/ih/decisions/fulltext/pdf/2020/paul-hirtle-13553692-sept2019-penalty.pdf

College of Nurses of Ontario. (2019b). *Ethics*. https://www.cno.org/globalassets/docs/prac/41034_ethics.pdf

College of Nurses of Ontario. (2020a). *About the college of nurses of Ontario*. https://www.cno.org/en/what-is-cno/

College of Nurses of Ontario. (2020b). *Paul Hirtle, 13553692*. https://www.cno.org/en/learn-about-standards-guidelines/magazines-newsletters/the-standard/summarized-decisions/june-2020/paul-hirtle-13553692/

College of Nurses of Ontario. (2021). *Supporting learners*. https://www.cno.org/en/learn-about-standards-guidelines/educational-tools/ask-practice/supporting-learners/

College of Registered Nurses of Manitoba. (2018). *Practice direction: Practice expectation for RNs*. https://www.crnm.mb.ca/uploads/document/document_file_239.pdf?t=1529682107

Forrest, K. D., & Miller, R. L. (2008). Procedural justice in the college classroom. *Psychology Teacher Network*, 18(1). https://www.apa.org/ed/precollege/ptn/2008/03/issue.pdf

Granger (litigation guardian of), v. Ottawa General Hospital, [1996] OJ 2129.

Hardcastle, L. (2019). *Introduction to health law in Canada*. Emond.

Harelkin v. University of Regina, CanLII 18 (SCC), [1979] 2 SCR 561.

Huscroft, G. (2012). From natural justice to fairness – Thresholds, content, and the role of judicial review. In C. Flood & L. Sossin (Eds.), *Administrative law in context*. Emond Montgomery. https://ssrn.com/abstract=2013253

Miller, L. (2020). Understanding regulatory, legislative, and credentialling requirements in Canada. In E. Staples, R. Pilon, & R. A. Hannon (Eds.), *Canadian perspectives on advanced practice nursing*, (2nd ed., pp. 86–98). Canadian Scholars.

Nelson, E., & Ogbogu, U. (2018). *Law for healthcare providers*. LexisNexis.

Patton, C. W., & Lewallen, L. P. (2015). Legal issues in clinical nursing education. *Nurse Educator, 40*(3), 124–128. https://doi.org/10.1097/NNE.0000000000000122

Regulated Health Professions Act, RSO 1991, c 18.

Schiller, C. (2015). Self-regulation of the nursing profession: Focus on four Canadian provinces. *Journal of Nursing Education and Practice, 5*(2), 95–106. https://doi.org/10.5430/jnep.v5n1p95

Schiller, C. (2020). *The space to make mistakes: Allocating responsibility and accountability for nursing student-committed medication errors* [Doctoral dissertation, University of Northern British Columbia]. CORE. https://core.ac.uk/download/pdf/343652368.pdf

Yao v. University of Saskatchewan, 2014 SKQB 184.

APPENDIX

The Canadian Association of Schools of Nursing supports the following CI competencies

1. **Enacts the educational role and responsibilities of clinical nursing instructors in preparing baccalaureate nursing students for entry into the profession.**

Indicators
- Recognizes that the clinical instructor role is an educational role that requires the effective use of teaching and learning principles and strategies.
- Articulates the need for clinical instructors to understand the curriculum and how the objectives of the clinical course align with the curriculum.
- Articulates a clear understanding of the objectives and assessment modalities of the clinical course.
- Recognizes that the clinical instructor's role is to facilitate the student's progress in meeting the learning objectives.
- Identifies their own learning needs and seeks appropriate information about educational program expectations, the curriculum, clinical course and the agency.
- Collaborates effectively with faculty in the delivery of a clinical course.
- Describes the responsibilities of the clinical instructor in preparing the student for a clinical practice setting.
- Collaborates effectively with the service agency's administration and staff when teaching nursing students.
- Differentiates between the role of the preceptor, the practice nurse and the clinical instructor.

2. **Integrates ethical principles and understands legal obligations of a clinical instructor.**

Indicators
- Articulates key ethical principles that guide clinical instructing including respecting the confidentiality of student, patient and agency data, and demonstrating fairness and integrity.
- Models the integration of ethical principles and ethical care delivery to students and guides students in ethical care delivery.
- Practices according to ethical, legal and professional standards of the profession.
- Understands and respects policies and processes for evaluating and grading students, as well as the appeals processes of the educational institution.
- Identifies relevant resources for clinical instructors.

3. Creates a positive learning environment for nursing students

   Indicators
   - Collaborates with students to establish respectful and supportive relationships.
   - Facilitates student learning through mentorship and coaching.
   - Explains how a clinical practice course is a learning experience and that students' knowledge and skill development is progressive
   - Identifies personal biases and avoids premature judgements regarding students' performance.
   - Utilizes effective communication strategies when interacting with agency and partner organization staff, patients/clients, and families to create a supportive environment for student learning.
   - Describes diverse teaching and learning styles, adult education principles, the development of a lesson plan, and self-directed learning approaches.
   - Applies learning strategies that reflect adult education principles, facilitates self-directed learning, and takes into account students' learning styles.

4. Applies key theoretical principles of clinical instructing in acute care settings

   Indicators
   - Utilizes the learning objectives of the clinical course to support student learning.
   - Describes key considerations that guide effective patient assignments in an acute care setting.
   - Integrates best practices in leading pre-clinical and post-clinical conferences.
   - Describes a typical day instructing students and the clinical learning activities that facilitate students' progress in meeting the course objectives.
   - Provides timely and effective feedback to students that facilitates their progress in meeting the course objectives.
   - Assesses students' comprehension and knowledge acquisition in the clinical setting.
   - Sets priorities when working with multiple learners of varying abilities.
   - Utilizes constructive strategies to address common clinical learning challenges.
   - Facilitates the development of learner reflexivity.

5. Applies key theoretical principles of clinical instructing in public health and community settings

   Indicators
   - Liaises with community resources and agencies.
   - Utilizes best practices in conducting group learning sessions to facilitate meeting course objectives.
   - Manages distance supervision of multiple learners and multiple sites effectively.
   - Sets priorities when communicating with preceptors, learners and agencies.
   - Explains and justifies the selection of site visits vs telephone support vs email support.
   - Utilizes constructive strategies to address common clinical learning challenges.

6. Analyzes and evaluates nursing students' clinical knowledge and skills

Indicators

- Uses a variety of methods to observe and analyze nursing students' level of clinical knowledge and skills throughout a clinical placement.
- Questions students respectfully and skillfully to assess preparation and knowledge.
- Identifies common challenges of clinical instructing that need to be addressed including the underperforming or failing student, behavioural and/or ethical issues among students, and inadequate or inappropriate preparation for clinical practice.
- Recognizes and responds to differences in learning pace and styles.
- Applies constructive strategies that enable positive learning experiences and outcomes in response to common student issues during a clinical placement.
- Develops and monitors learning plans for students to address knowledge gaps and/or performance issues.
- Assesses potentially problematic behaviours of students during a clinical placement and addresses these in a timely and constructive manner.
- Formulates an evaluation of the students' achievement of the learning objectives of the clinical course.
- Utilizes effective communication strategies to deliver evaluation results to students in a supportive and respectful manner.

INDEX

Note: Figures are indicated by page numbers in italics

A

academic appeal, 142–43, 144–47
acute care, 4, 54
acute care placements: about, 54, 83; access to charting and patient information, 58–59, 64; addressing student concerns, fears, and anxieties, 61; background and history, 54–55; badge attachment of do's and don'ts, 65–66, *66*; communication, 74; conflict, 76–77; creating an organized routine, 67, 67–68; day planners, time sheets, and nurse's brain, *68*, 68; debriefing, 79–80; documentation, 71; evaluation, 81–82; familiarity with medications, diagnoses, skills, and procedures, 69; filling down time, 72–73; fitting into, 59; getting to know students, 60; goal setting, 81; handling errors, 75–76; handling uncertainties, 73–78; interprofessional collaboration, 61–62; learning opportunities beyond task completion, 72; managing students' external factors, 57; orientation, *55–56*, 55–57, 61; patient assignments, 63–65; patient deterioration, 73–74; patient logs and care plans, 70; personalized pocket reference tools, 69; post-conferences, 78–79, *79*; preceptors and staff nurses, 64, 73, 77; pre-conferences, 63; professional conduct, 62; reflection-in-action, 77–78; reflection-on-action, 78; reflective journaling, 82; setting expectations, 57–58, 62, 64, 82; storytelling, 80–81; students as pre-service professionals, 65; Three Great Things activity, 82; travel to placement, 57; wrapping up, 78–81
adult education, 30–31. *See also* pedagogy
affective domain, 120
Alexander, G. K., 101
Almalkawi, I., 128
Al Shahrani, Y., 61
ambiguity, role, 107
ambulatory care movement, 4
andragogy, 30–31. *See also* pedagogy

anecdotal notes, 122
appeal, academic, 142–43, 144–47
Appeals Committee, 145–46
apprenticeship model (hospital-based training), 3, 5, 6, 7, 10, 14
approachability, 17
articulation, 46, 47
assessment and evaluation: about, 116, 130–31; academic appeal and, 142–43, 144–47; acute care placements, 81–82; assessment overview, 118–22; background, 116–17; community health placements, 92, 100, 108; and course outcomes and requirements, 120; data collection and performance analysis approaches, 122–23; dealing with student performance issues, 142–43; definitions, 117; evaluation process overview, 118, *118*; feedback, 17, 19–20, 48, 123–24, *124*, *125*; formal clinical evaluation tools, *127*, 127–28; formative evaluation, 122–26; formative vs. summative evaluation, 117, *117*; grading, 128, *129*; implications for clinical instructors, 130; mid-course evaluation, 125; and personal biases, values, and assumptions, 34–35, 119; personal learning plans and, 121, *122*, 128; reflection journaling and, 82; remediation plan (learning contract) and, 125–26, *126*, 143, 145; of students' clinical learning needs, 120–21; summative evaluation, 127–30; Three Great Things activity, 82; unsuccessful students, 129–30
assignments: patient assignments, 63–65; written clinical assignments, 123
assumptions, 119
Athabasca University, 16
attitude, supportive, 16
auditory learners, 30
autonomy, 58, 107

B

badge attachment, of do's and don'ts, 65–66, *66*
balance theory, 82
Bandura, A., 82

Benner, Patricia, 9, 44, 67, 72, 77
bias, 34–35, 119
big picture, difficulties seeing, 49
Bjekić, D., 36
Bloom's taxonomy, 32, *32*
Boyer, L., 44
Bristol, T., 72
British Columbia College of Nurses and Midwives (BCCNM): *Ethical Practice Professional Standard*, 136; regulatory supervision standard, 137, 138; scope of practice and, 137
Bussard, M., 70

C

Cahill, M., 70
Canadian Association of Schools of Nursing (CASN): Canadian Nurse Educator Institute, 16; competencies for clinical instructors, 150–52; *Entry-to-Practice Public Health Nursing Competencies for Undergraduate Nursing Education*, 92; on getting to know students, 60
Canadian Council of Practical Nurse Regulators: *Code of Ethics for Licensed Practical Nurses*, 136
Canadian Institutes of Health Research (CIHR), 54
Canadian Interprofessional Health Collaborative (CIHC), 61
Canadian Medical Association: Weir Report, 3
Canadian Nurse Educator Institute, 16
Canadian Nurses Association (CNA): *Code of Ethics for Registered Nurses*, 95, 136; *Framework for the Practice of Registered Nurses in Canada*, 57; Weir Report, 3
Canadian Nurses Protection Society: Supplementary Protection Program, 138
care plans, 70
Carnegie Foundation, 4
charting and patient information, access to, 58–59, 64
checklists, 122
Chickering, A. W., 29, 123
civil law, 139–41; about, 139; mitigating risks, 140–41; negligence, 139–40
clarity, 35
clinical assignments, 123
clinical competence, 44. *See also* clinical expertise; clinical judgement and reasoning
clinical decision-making, 42. *See also* clinical judgement and reasoning

clinical education. *See* clinical teaching
clinical evaluation, 117. *See also* assessment and evaluation
clinical expertise, 15. *See also* clinical competence; clinical judgement and reasoning
clinical fatigue, 79
clinical hours: for community health placements, 92, 98; variation across programs, 120
clinical instructors (CIs): about, 14, 22; approachability, 17; background and history, 5–6, 14–15; characteristics of, 15–17; clinical and instructional expertise, 15–16; as clinical supervisor, 98–99; as coach and mentor, 100–101; as collaborator, 101; communication with, 17; in community health placements, 5, 98–101; competencies for, 150–52; evaluating students and, 130; increased enrolments and, 7; indirect supervision by, 5; instructor-clinical collaborations, 21–22; instructor-faculty collaborations, 21; instructor-program collaborations, 21; instructor-student collaborations, 19–20; passion for the profession, 17; personal biases, values, and assumptions, 34–35, 119; and program and course curricula, 18–19; role modelling by, 16–17, 46, 100–101; strategies for student-teacher relationships, 27–29; student-student collaborations and, 20; supervisory expectations, 5; supportive attitude, 16; teaching role, 6. *See also* pedagogy
clinical judgement and reasoning: about, 41, 50; clinical competence and, 44; clinical teaching for, 45–47; cognitive strategies for, 42; definitions, 9–10, 41–42; development during training, 44, *45*; difficulties and remediation strategies, 48, *48*–49; health assessment and, 43; knowledge and, 42–43; nurse's background and, 43; practical points for effective supervision, 47–48; research on and evidence for, 42–43
clinical placements, diversification of, 6. *See also* acute care placements; clinical teaching; community health placements
clinical reasoning. *See* clinical judgement and reasoning
clinical skills, 7–10; cognitive skills, 8–10, 120; providing students with information about, 69; psychomotor skills, 120; relational skills, 8; task-based skills, 7–8

clinical supervisor role, 98–99. *See also* clinical instructors
clinical teaching (practice-based learning): about, 2, 10; apprenticeship model (hospital-based training), 3, 5, 6, 7, 10, 14; background and history, 3–5; clinical skill development, 7–10; diversification of, 6–7; evolution of clinical instructor role, 5–6, 14–15; Hall Commission Report, 4; health care complexity and, 4; university education for nurses and, 3, 5, 6, 14–15, 54, 91. *See also* acute care placements; assessment and evaluation; clinical instructors; clinical judgement and reasoning; community health placements; legal and ethical issues; pedagogy
coaching, 46, 100–101. *See also* feedback
Code Blue, 73–74
code of ethics, 95, 136
cognitive companionship, 45–47
cognitive skills, 8–10, 120
Cohen, B. E., 92
collaboration, 19–22; in community health placements, 101, 106–7; instructor-clinical, 21–22; instructor-faculty, 21; instructor-program, 21; instructor-student, 19–20, 125; interprofessional, 61–62; intersectoral, 96; student-student, 20
College of Nurses of Ontario (CNO): disciplinary examples, 136; *Ethics Practice Standard*, 136; *Practice standard: Documentation*, 71; professional standards practice standard, 136; regulatory guidance for student supervision, 137
communication: in acute care placements, 74; clinical instructors and, 17; SBAR (situation, background, assessment, and recommendation) communication, 74, 75; storytelling, 80–81; strategies for, 35–36; student performance concerns and, 142–43
community, entering into, 104
community health placements: about, 90, 108–9; autonomy, self-direction, and role ambiguity, 107; background and history, 91; challenges and strategies, 106–8; client-centred, strength-based, and relational practice, 94; clinical hours, 92, 98; clinical instructor roles, 5, 98–101; clinical supervisor role, 98–99; coaching and mentoring, 100–101; collaborative partnerships, 101, 106–7; conferences with students, 96–97, 98; documentation, 97; entering the community, 104; entry-to-practice competencies, 92; ethical frameworks for, 95; evaluation, 92, 100, 108; and health and social inequalities, 95; indirect supervision, 5, 98; intersectoral collaborations, 96; involving students in teaching strategies, 105; learning context, 93–97; lesson plans, 102; new perspectives on clients/patients, 93; non-structured/minimally structured learning environments, 93; nursing career choice and, 97; orientation, 103–4; practice standards, 94; safety, 107; self and group reflection, 104; service-learning, 105; student projects, 95–96, 106; teaching and learning strategies, 102–6; team-based learning, 105; time limitations and course outcomes, 108; traditional and non-traditional settings, 91–92
compassion, 35
competence, clinical, 44. *See also* clinical expertise; clinical judgement and reasoning
competencies: for clinical instructors, 150–52; entry-to-practice for community and public health nursing, 92
complaints and discipline, 136, 138
conferences: in community health placements, 96–97, 98; post-conferences, 78–79, 79; pre-conferences, 63
confidentiality and privacy, 62, 68, 97, 123, 136
conflict, 76–77
connection, in teacher-student relationship, 29
contact plans, 21
continuing education, for instructional expertise, 16
contract, learning (remediation plan), 125–26, *126*, 143, 145
courses: familiarity with curricula, outcomes, and requirements, 18–19, 120; lesson plans, 31–33, 102; syllabus, 142
COVID-19 pandemic, 106, 120–21
Creative Clinical Teaching in the Health Professions (Melrose, Park, and Perry), 16
criminal law, 139
criterion-referenced evaluation, 128
critical social theory, 105
critical thinking, 9, 41, 42, 63, 120. *See also* clinical judgement and reasoning
culture, unit, 59
curricula/curriculum, 18–19

D

Dafogianni, C., 80–81
Dalhousie University, 91
data collection: for formative evaluation, 122–23; student difficulties with and remediation strategies, 48
day planners, 68, *68*
DeBrew, J. K., 129
debriefing, 79–80
decision-making, clinical, 42. *See also* clinical judgement and reasoning
demeanour, approachable, 17
Dewey, J., 77
diagnoses, providing students with information about, 69
direct observation, 122
discipline and complaints, 136, 138
Doane, H. G., 8
documentation, 71, 97. *See also* charting and patient information
down time, filling, 72–73

E

education and educational institutions, 141–47; about, 141; academic appeal, 142–43, 144–47; continuing education for instructional expertise, 16; educational support for students, 27; familiarity with curricula, outcomes, and requirements, 18–19, 120; familiarity with policies and procedures, 142; learning contract (remediation plan), 125–26, *126*, 143, 145; lesson plans, 31–33, 102; pre-term preparations, 141; student performance concerns, 142–43; syllabus, 142. *See also* nursing education; pedagogy
emotions: emotional support, 27; expressivity and sensitivity, 36
empathy, 34–35
empowerment, 36
entry-to-practice competencies, 92
environmental management, 107
equality, 80
errors, handling, 75–76
Estepp, C. M., 28, 29
Esteves, L. S. F., 98
ethical codes and frameworks, 95, 136. *See also* legal and ethical issues
evaluation. *See* assessment and evaluation
expectations, setting, 57–58, 62, 64, 82, 120, 142, 143
expertise, 15–16
exploration, 47
external conflict, 77
external factors, managing, 57
Ezhova, I., 94, 101

F

faculty, collaborations with, 21
failure to fail, 130
Fainstad, T. L., 119
fatigue, clinical, 79
feedback: about, 48, 81; approachability and, 17; coaching and, 46, 100–101; examples of supportive comments, *124*; general principles, 123–24; instructor-student collaborations and, 19–20; ongoing feedback, 125; for preceptors, 73; reflective journaling and, 82; Three Great Things activity and, 82. *See also* formative evaluation
Flexner Report, 3
Fonteyn, M. E., 70
formative evaluation, 122–26; about, 117, 122; data collection and performance analysis approaches, 122–23; feedback, 17, 19–20, 48, 123–24, *124*, 125; mid-course evaluation, 125; remediation plan (learning contract), 125–26, *126*, 143, 145; vs. summative evaluation, *117*. *See also* assessment and evaluation
Framework for Ethical Deliberation and Decision-Making in Public Health, 95

G

Gamson, Z. F., 29, 123
Gantt chart, 102, *103*
Ghasemi, M. R., 105
goal setting, 81, 121
Gottman, J. M., 82
grading, 128, *129*
Granger (Litigation Guardian of) v. Ottawa General Hospital [1996], 140
Gregory, D., 92
group dynamics, 20, *21*, 77, 99. *See also* team-based learning
group projects, student, 95–96, 106

H

Hall Commission Report, 4
health assessment, 43
health inequalities, 95
health promotion, 100–101
Health Protection and Promotion Act (Ontario), 91
Henneman, E. A., 75
Heydari, A., 27
home health. *See* community health placements
hospital-based training (apprenticeship model), 3, 5, 6, 7, 10, 14
hours. *See* clinical hours
Hughes, L. J., 130
hypotheses generation and validation, 42, 47, 49

I

ID badge, attachment of do's and don'ts, 65–66, 66
Indigenous Peoples, 43, 104
indirect supervision, 5, 98
inequalities, health and social, 95
informal data, 123
instructional expertise, 15–16
instructor-clinical collaborations, 21–22
instructor-faculty collaborations, 21
instructor-program collaborations, 21
instructor-student collaborations, 19–20, 125
insurance, 138, 141
internal conflict, 77
interprofessional collaborations, 61–62. *See also* intersectoral collaborations
interprofessional presentations, 79
intersectoral collaborations, 96. *See also* interprofessional collaborations
intuition, 42
invitational education theory, 28
Ironside, P. M., 72

J

Jensen, M., 20, *21*
Johns, Ethel, 91
journal club activity, 79
journaling, reflective, 82
judgement. *See* assessment and evaluation; clinical judgement and reasoning
justice: natural justice, 145; social justice, 92, 95, 100–101

K

Keller, L. O., 108
kindness, pedagogy of, 34–35
kinesthetic learners, 30
knowledge, and decision-making, 42–43
Knowles, M. S., 30, 33
Kramer, M., 4

L

learning activities: about, 33; badge attachment of do's and don'ts, 65–66, *66*; day planners, time sheets, and nurse's brain, 68, *68*; interprofessional presentations, *79*; journal club, *79*; minute to win it, *79*; NCLEX-style questions, *79*; nursing handover, *79*; patient charts, 59; patient logs and care plans, 70; personalized pocket reference tools, 69; for post-conference, *79*; reflective journaling, 82; role-playing, 104; SBAR (situation, background, assessment, and recommendation) communication, 74, *75*; scavenger hunt, 56–57; shadow shift, 57; Three Great Things, 82; wayfinding, 56
learning contract (remediation plan), 125–26, *126*, 143, 145
learning outcomes, 31–32
learning plans, personal, 121, *122*, 128
learning styles, 29–30
legal and ethical issues: about, 134, 147; academic appeal, 142–43, 144–47; background and history, 135; civil law, 139–41; complaints and discipline, 136, 138; criminal law, 139; educational institution issues, 141–47; ethical codes and frameworks, 95, 136; familiarity with policies and procedures, 142; insurance, 138, 141; learning contract (remediation plan), 125–26, *126*, 143, 145; mitigating risks, 140–41; negligence, 139–40; nursing regulation in Canada, 135; pre-term preparations, 141; regulatory issues, 135–38; scope of practice, 137; standards of practice, 94, 135–36; student performance concerns, 142–43; student supervision, 137–38; syllabus, 142
Leighton, K., 116
lesson plans, 31–33; about, 31; for community health placements, 102; learning activities, 33; learning outcomes, 31–32; self-directed

learning, 33. *See also* learning activities; pedagogy
Lewallen, L. P., 129
Lin, F. Y., 76

M

MacDonald, J., 57
Mack Training School for Nurses, *2*, 3
Mamchur, C., 77
Matheney, R. V., 63
McGill University, 91
McGregor, A., 130
medical-surgical units, acute, 54
medications, providing students with information about, 69
Meeley, N. G., 100
Melrose, S., 58; *Creative Clinical Teaching in the Health Professions* (with Park and Perry), 16
mentoring, 100–101. *See also* coaching; modelling
minute to win it activity, 79
modelling, 16–17, 46, 100–101
Monteiro, S., 42
Murdoch, N. L., 61–62
Mussallem, Helen, 91
Myrick, F., 77

N

National Collaborating Centre for Determinants of Health (NCCDH), 95
natural justice, 145
NCLEX-style questions, 79
negligence, 139–40
networking, 19, 21. *See also* collaboration
Nicholson, Helen F., 63
Noland, C., 75
norm-referenced evaluation, 128
Nugent, O., 130
nurses and nursing: career choices, 97; code of ethics, 95, 136; complaints and discipline, 136, 138; development throughout career, 44; regulation in Canada, 135; scope of practice, 137; socialization into nursing culture, 59; standards of practice, 94, 135–36; student supervision by, 137–38; working with in acute care placements, 64, 73, 77. *See also* nursing education
nurse's brain, 68, *68*
nursing education: apprenticeship model (hospital-based training), 3, 5, 6, 7, 10, 14; clinical instructor role, 5–6; Hall Commission Report and, 4; health care complexity and, 4; historical overview, 3–5; increased enrolments, 7; in universities, 3, 5, 6, 14–15, 54, 91. *See also* acute care placements; assessment and evaluation; clinical instructors; clinical judgement and reasoning; clinical teaching; community health placements; education and educational institutions; learning activities; legal and ethical issues; pedagogy
nursing handover activity, 79

O

observation, direct, 122
Oermann, M. H., 6, 118–19
Ontario, 91, 137
open educational resources (OERs), 16
orientation, 19, *55–56*, 55–57, 61, 103–4
outcomes, learning, 31–32

P

Park, C.: *Creative Clinical Teaching in the Health Professions* (with Melrose and Perry), 16
passion, for profession, 17
patients: access to patient information and charting, 58–59, 64; client-centred, strength-based, and relational practice, 94; in community health placements, 93; confidentiality and privacy, 62, 68, 97; deterioration and high acuity, 73–74; patient assignments, 63–65; patient logs, 70
pedagogy: about, 26, 36–37; adult education and, 30–31; background and history, 26; communication strategies, 35–36; connecting with students, 29; involving students in teaching strategies, 105; of kindness, 34–35; learning activities, 33; learning outcomes, 31–32; lesson plans, 31–33, 102; personal biases and premature judgement, 34–35, 119; respect and, 28; self-directed learning, 33; service-learning, 105; strategies for supporting students, 27–28; and teaching and learning styles, 29–30; team-based learning, 105. *See also* assessment and evaluation; education and educational institutions; learning activities; nursing education
Peplau, Hildegarde, 8

Perry, B.: *Creative Clinical Teaching in the Health Professions* (with Melrose and Park), 16
personal learning plans, 121, *122*, 128
placements, diversification of, 6. *See also* acute care placements; clinical teaching; community health placements
planner, day, 68, *68*
pocket reference tools, personalized, 69
policies and procedures (P&P), 142
post-conferences, 78–79, *79*
practice-based learning. *See* clinical teaching
practice standards, 94, 135–36
practicums. *See* clinical teaching
preceptors, 73, 77
pre-conferences, 63
presentations, interprofessional, 79
pre-service professionals, 65
primary care. *See* community health placements
prioritizing, difficulties with, 49
privacy and confidentiality, 62, 68, 97, 123, 136
problem solving, 8–9
procedures, providing students with information about, 69
professional conduct, 62
professional liability protection, 141
program curricula, 18
progression plan (remediation plan, learning contract), 125–26, *126*, 143, 145
psychomotor skills, 120
Public Health Agency of Canada (PHAC): entry-to-practice competencies and, 92; *Framework for Ethical Deliberation and Decision-Making in Public Health*, 95
public health nursing, 91. *See also* community health placements
Purkey, W. W., 28

R

reality shock, 4
reasoning. *See* clinical judgement and reasoning
reflection: about, 46–47; for community health placements, 104; journaling, 82; for personal biases, values, and assumptions, 34–35, 119; reflection-in-action, 77–78; reflection-on-action, 78; Three Great Things activity, 82
Registered Nurses' Association of Ontario: Legal Assistance Program, 138
Regulated Health Professions Act (Ontario), 137

regulatory colleges, 135
regulatory issues, 135–38; complaints and discipline, 136, 138; ethical codes and frameworks, 95, 136; nursing regulation in Canada, 135; scope of practice, 137; standards of practice, 94, 135–36; student supervision, 137–38
relational inquiry, 8
relational practice, 94
relational skills, 8
relevant cues, 43, 47, 48
remediation plan (learning contract), 125–26, *126*, 143, 145
respect, 28
risks, mitigating, 140–41
Roberts, T. G., 28, 29
role ambiguity, 107
role modelling, 16–17, 46, 100–101
role-playing, 74, 104
Rolfe, G., 78
routine, creating for students, 67, 67–68
rural and remote community health nursing. *See* community health placements

S

safety, 107
salience, sense of, 9
SARS health crisis, 92
SBAR (situation, background, assessment, and recommendation) communication, 74, *75*
scaffolding, 46
scavenger hunts, 56–57
Schon, D., 77
scope of practice, 137
Sedlak, C. A., 70
self-direction, 33, 107
self-reflection. *See* reflection
service for training, 14. *See also* apprenticeship model
service-learning, 105
shadow shifts, 57
signature, student, 71
skills. *See* clinical skills
Smith, P. M., 54
social determinants of health, 93, 106
socialization, into nursing culture, 59
social justice, 92, 95, 100–101
social learning theory, 82
social support, 28
Socratic questioning, 80

spare time, filling, 72–73
standards of practice, 94, 135–36
Steffy, M. L., 98
storytelling, 80–81
strength-based approaches, 94
students: academic appeal, 142–43, 144–47; addressing concerns, fears, and anxieties of, 61; assessing clinical learning needs of, 120–21; connecting with and getting to know, 29, 60; contact plans, 21; errors by, 75–76; group projects, 95–96, 106; instructor-student collaborations, 19–20; interprofessional collaborations, 61–62; involving in teaching strategies, 105; managing external factors of, 57; as pre-service professionals, 65; professional conduct and, 62; respect and, 28; setting placement expectations, 57–58; signatures, 71; student-student collaborations, 20; supporting students, 27–28; travel to clinical placements, 57, 107; unsuccessful students, 129–30. *See also* acute care placements; assessment and evaluation; clinical judgement and reasoning; clinical teaching; community health placements; nursing education
summative evaluation, 127–30; about, 117, 127; formal clinical evaluation tools, *127*, 127–28; vs. formative evaluation, *117*; grading, 128, *129*; implications for clinical instructor, 130; unsuccessful students, 129–30. *See also* assessment and evaluation
supervision: in community health placements, 98–99; expectations for clinical instructors, 5; indirect supervision, 5, 98; regulatory guidance for, 137–38
support: attitude and, 16; educational support, 27; emotional support, 27; for learning clinical judgement and reasoning, 47–48; for preceptors, 73; social support, 28
Sybing, R., 29
syllabus, 142

T

Tanner, C. A., 9–10, 41, 42, 43, 70, *103*
task-based skills, 7–8
task completion, 72
teaching: by clinical instructors, 6; teaching and learning styles, 29–30. *See also* clinical teaching; education and educational institutions; learning activities; pedagogy
team-based learning, 105. *See also* group dynamics
Three Great Things activity, 82
time limitations, 108
time sheets, 68
Toews, A. J., 80
travel, to clinical placement, 57, 107
Travelbee, Joyce, 8
trust, 34
Tuckman, B., 20, *21*, 77

U

university education, for nursing, 3, 5, 6, 14–15, 54, 91
University of Alberta, 91
University of British Columbia (UBC), 3, 65, 91
University of Montreal, 91
University of Toronto, 54, 91
University of Western Ontario, 91

V

Valaitis, R. K., 101
values, personal, 119
Varcoe, C., 8
VARK (visual, auditory, reading/writing, and kinesthetic) Model, of student learning, 29–30
visual learners, 29–30

W

Watson, Jean, 8
wayfinding, 56
Weir, G., 3

Manufactured by Amazon.ca
Acheson, AB